Bound To Be Free

The Liberating Power of Prison Yoga

Rev. Sandra Kumari de Sachy, Ed.D.

Library of Congress Cataloging in Publication Data

De Sachy, Sandra Kumari, 1942-
Bound to be free: the liberating power of prison yoga
based on the teachings of Sri Swami Satchidananda : featuring
his prison yoga talks / by Sandra Kumari de Sachy.

p. cm.

ISBN 978-0-932040-65-7

1. Yoga. 2. Prisoners--Religious life. 3. Satchidananda, Swami,
1914-2002. I. Satchidananda, Swami, 1914-2002. II. Title.

BL1238.54.D47 2009
294.5'4360883656--dc22
                    2009028552

Integral Yoga® Publications
Satchidananda Ashram–Yogaville
108 Yogaville Way
Buckingham, Virginia 23921 USA

Dedication

This book is dedicated to our beloved spiritual master, Sri Swami Satchidananda, whose love, compassion and wisdom knows no bounds; to the Yoga teachers who are serving in prison, opening their hearts and minds to those who are often scorned; to prison volunteers who lovingly share their expertise in many areas; to prison staff members who support programs that offer inmates opportunities for self-growth; and, of course, to the prisoners, themselves, who willingly and generously shared their stories and insights and welcomed me so warmly into their world.

Acknowledgments

Kudos to Maitreyi Villaman. She conceived the idea for the book and researched Swami Satchidananda's service in prisons; her passion and abundant creative energy triggered the release of my own creative impulse; to Swami Murugananda, manager of the Satchidananda Ashram-Yogaville library and creator of the SASTRI Program, an archive of Sri Swami Satchidananda's talks, *Integral Yoga Magazine* articles and other Integral Yoga writings and publications; to Dr. Prem Anjali, project manager, for her tireless support and commitment to the dissemination of the Integral Yoga teachings; to Peter Petronio for creating a book cover that compellingly illustrates the power of Prison Yoga; to Anand Shiva Herve for the graphic design and layout of the interior of the book; to Kalyani Neuman and Swami Hamsananda for their dedication and excellent editing skills; to Kristofer Marsh and Abhaya Thiele for proofing; to Swami Priyaananda, manager of the Satchidananda Archives; to my husband, Snehan, for sharing his formidable critical skills; to all those who contributed financially and creatively to this project; and special thanks to Satish and Veena Daryanani, the Harry Wadhwani family, Purusha Carves and *Integral Yoga Magazine* donors for underwriting this project.

Freedom XIV

An orator said, "Speak to us of Freedom."

And he answered:

"At the city gate and by your fireside I have seen you prostrate yourself
and worship your own freedom,

even as slaves humble themselves before a tyrant and praise him though
he slays them.

Ay, in the grove of the temple and in the shadow of the citadel I have seen
the freest among you wear their freedom as a yoke and a handcuff.

And my heart bled within me; for you can only be free when even the
desire of seeking freedom becomes a harness to you, and when you
cease to speak of freedom as a goal and a fulfillment.

You shall be free indeed when your days are not without a care nor your
nights without a want and a grief, but rather when these things girdle
your life and yet you rise above them naked and unbound.

And how shall you rise beyond your days and nights unless you break
the chains which you at the dawn of your understanding have fastened
around your noon hour?

In truth that which you call freedom is the strongest of these chains,
though its links glitter in the sun and dazzle the eyes.

And what is it but fragments of your own self you would discard that you
may become free?

If it is an unjust law you would abolish, that law was written with your
own hand upon your own forehead.

You cannot erase it by burning your law books nor by washing the
foreheads of your judges, though you pour the sea upon them.

And if it is a despot you would dethrone, see first that his throne erected
within you is destroyed.

For how can a tyrant rule the free and the proud, but for a tyranny in
their own freedom and a shame in their won pride?

And if it is a care you would cast off, that care has been chosen by you
rather than imposed upon you.

And if it is a fear you would dispel, the seat of that fear is in your heart
and not in the hand of the feared.

Verily all things move within your being in constant half embrace, the
desired and the dreaded, the repugnant and the cherished, the pursued
and that which you would escape.

These things move within you as lights and shadows in pairs that cling.

And when the shadow fades and is no more, the light that lingers
becomes a shadow to another light.

And thus your freedom when it loses its fetters becomes itself the fetter of
a greater freedom." –Khalil Gibran

Contents

Introduction

We citizens of the United States think of our country as the land of the free. We're very proud of our democratic heritage and our constitutional rights. When we feel that our freedom is compromised, we can and do speak out or take action. But I wonder how many of us take the time to think deeply about a privilege that we, often, take for granted. How many ask themselves: What is freedom, really? Is it an attribute embraced by a particular society? An inalienable right guaranteed by law? A political or social property that can be conferred or revoked? A moral principle?

Of course, freedom is all of the above. But *true* freedom is more, much more than a socio-political guarantee of rights. In fact, when social or political freedom is informed by ignorance rather than by wisdom, then what you really have is *freedumb,* as my spiritual teacher, Sri Swami Satchidananda, used to say. On the deepest level of our being, on the level of wisdom and self-knowledge, freedom is not a quality that can be given to or taken away from us. From the spiritual perspective, freedom is an inner experience that is not contingent upon any external force. We can be free in any and every circumstance—*literally.* The afflicted, the oppressed, the sufferers, the exploited, the downtrodden, the condemned on death row can all be free without intervention from any outside source. What's more, they—and we—can be free right now, at this very moment. It's a fact. Whether we know it or not, it's inevitable: each and every one of us is bound to be free.

Bound to be free. A pun, yes, even an oxymoron if you think of freedom as an attribute that must be earned or fought for, something out there, a legal or moral privilege that once attained must be sustained. In that case, how can we be free if we're limited, restrained or confined? On the other hand, if you shift your perspective from the external to the internal world, you will eventually discover that on the deepest, most authentic level of being, *we are always free,* in any circumstance, under any condition, *even in prison.* Yes, we are always free to take responsibility for our thoughts, our actions and reactions. We are always free to embrace every situation as an opportunity to grow, an opportunity to evolve, to experience our full human potential. We are always free to choose love instead of hatred.

It is in this sense, that we are bound to be free. For the term "bound" also means to move by leaps, to spring forward, literally and figuratively. If you have the eyes to see, you will notice that we're all moving, sometimes by leaps and bounds and sometimes by stops and starts, toward the realization that we are, in the core of our being and by our very nature, free spirits. Of course, it may seem cavalier or even cruel to say that people who are imprisoned are essentially free. But, again, I'm talking about real freedom. Real freedom is freedom from suffering, and this freedom is not limited by status or circumstance or physical boundaries. It's a state of mind, an attitude.

A remarkable example of someone who remained totally free while enslaved in the midst of unquestionably horrific conditions is the late Victor Frankl, an eminent and innovative psychiatrist and neurologist. An Austrian Jew, Frankl spent years during World War II in four Nazi death camps, a witness to and victim of unspeakable atrocities perpetrated against millions by a ruthless group of his fellow Europeans. Taken against his will, enslaved, thought of and treated as subhuman, Frankl retained his optimism and faith. He never saw himself as his captors saw him, as a victim. In his mind, he was free. Why? Because he knew that true freedom is a state of mind. In his inspired and inspiring book, *Man's Search for Meaning*, Victor Frankl wrote, "Everything can be taken from a man but . . . the last of the human freedoms—to choose one's attitude in any given set of circumstances, to choose one's own way."

Victor Frankl's attitude reflects the nature of his liberated mind, and a liberated mind, a mind grounded in real freedom, is free from suffering. You may be incarcerated for a crime that you have or have not committed, you may be a political prisoner whose civil rights have been taken away, or you may be a slave labor camp survivor who witnessed and experienced the darkest side of human nature; but, like Victor Frankl, you can remain free even in the face of extreme physical and psychological challenges. What does it take? Obviously, it takes courage and will, hope and optimism. But, on an even more subtle level, it takes a pure and refined ego, an ego that does our bidding rather than an ego that rules us. And how can we develop such an ego? This is where the "C" word comes in: *commitment*. We must commit ourselves to a process of self-transformation, to a course of action that requires mindfulness, as well as vigilant self-analysis and self-correction.

To be truly free, that is to say, to be always peaceful, we must extricate ourselves from the domination of a tyrannical ego that compels us to satisfy its self-serving desires. In the yogic teachings, this process of cleansing, of refining the ego is called *tapasya*, a Sanskrit word that means, literally, "burning." Symbolically, you are burning up your attachments, your mind and your intellect in order to purify them. The image used to illustrate this process is that of a fritter. Like a fritter that needs to be fully fried in order to be edible and tasty, we too must be fried in the hot oil of our life experiences. And if we jump out before we're fully cooked? We'll be half-baked and, inevitably, we will have to be fried some more. As Sri Swami Satchidananda used to say, if you want to experience real freedom, total liberation, you must accept any hardship or pain without inflicting the same on others. Ultimately, you must tell the ego: "E, go!" Through this commitment and with the help of the Yoga teachings and practices, the process of refinement, *tapasya*, not only becomes understandable and bearable, but–believe it or not–it also becomes welcome. The result: you are no longer a slave of the ego; you become a liberated soul, a *jivanmukta*.

As a matter of fact, according to the yogic philosophy, whether we consciously choose to refine our egos or not, this process is inevitable in the cosmic scheme of things. And, ultimately, at some point in our present life or in a future lifetime, we will awaken to the realization that we are slaves of the ego. Normally, this realization comes through great suffering, whether physical, emotional, or spiritual or a package deal that includes all three (à la

Saint John of the Cross's "dark night of the soul"). Yoga can play a vital role in helping us utilize suffering to refine the ego, transform the character and experience the bliss of total freedom. And the beauty of Yoga is that it isn't tied to a particular geographical location, population, or spiritual or philosophical tradition. As you will discover in this book, Yoga travels everywhere, including prisons and correctional centers all over the world. Indeed, for centuries, people have used the teachings and practices of Yoga to liberate themselves from the bondage that takes hold when the mind is filled with selfish, egoistic desires.

Essentially, this book illustrates how prison Yoga can help prisoners reform and rehabilitate themselves. At the same time, it offers a glimpse of how a renowned Yoga master and proponent of interfaith harmony, Sri Swami Satchidananda, or Gurudev, as his disciples call him, brought the teachings and the teachers of Integral Yoga into prisons so that inmates might have the opportunity to experience the liberating power of Yoga.

Chapter 1
The Swami Goes to Prison

*Years ago, I recognized my kinship with all living things, and I made
up my mind that I was not one bit better than the meanest on the earth.
I said then and I say now that while there is a lower class, I am in it;
while there is a criminal element, I am of it; while there is a soul in
prison, I am not free. —Eugene Debs*

Sri Gurudev Swami Satchidananda was born in South India
in 1914. After studying with many well-known yogis and spiritual
teachers, he found his guru, H. H. Sri Swami Sivananda Maharaj,
at the Divine Life Society in Rishikesh, India, in the spring of
1949. In July of the same year, he was initiated into the Holy
Order of *Sannyas*, becoming a renunciate, or *swami* in Sanskrit, the
ancient, classical Indian language. From 1952 to 1966, he served
in Sri Lanka; and in 1966, he was invited by filmmaker Conrad
Rooks to visit the United States. During his visit to the US, he
was beseeched to stay by the young Americans who were inspired
by his teachings and who were yearning for spiritual guidance.
Recognizing their sincerity and deep thirst for the yogic teachings,
Gurudev agreed to move to the US. He became a US citizen in
1976.

Constantly invited to share his teachings and wisdom, Gurudev
traveled far and wide to disseminate the ancient science of Yoga.
He was one of the first Yoga masters to make the yogic teachings
and practices available to eager students in the West. At Integral
Yoga *ashrams* and institutes, here and abroad, countless students
became and—more than 40 years after his arrival in the West—
continue to become certified Integral Yoga teachers.

Above all, Gurudev conveyed—in his teachings and in his
life—his realization of the unity that underlies the diversity of
creation. He saw the same consciousness in everyone, whoever
or wherever they were. Along with other like-minded clergy, he
created interfaith worship services and retreats. His vision of an
interfaith shrine, a shrine that would be dedicated to all faiths and
traditions, became reality in July of 1986 with the opening of the

Light Of Truth Universal Shrine (LOTUS) at Satchidananda Ashram-Yogaville in Buckingham, Virginia. After more than 35 years of service in the US, Gurudev entered *Mahasamadhi* (when an enlightened soul leaves the physical body) in August 2002.

Gurudev first began visiting prisons in Sri Lanka (then Ceylon) in the mid-1950s. His sojourn in Sri Lanka began at the close of 1952, when his guru, Sri Swami Sivananda Maharaj, sent him to the city of Trincomalee where one of his disciples, a female *sannyasin* (monk) also named Swami Satchidananda, and a group of devotees planned to start a branch of the Divine Life Society. The female Swami Satchidananda requested that her male namesake accompany her to Ceylon to start the organization there, because he was an excellent teacher and because Tamil, the language spoken by the local devotees, was his mother-tongue.

However, at that time, co-directing an *ashram* was the last thing Gurudev desired. He was content with his work, preferring to continue his meditation and seclusion in Rishikesh. To his guru, he expressed concern that he wasn't fit to co-direct an *ashram* and that there would be confusion in having two Swami Satchidanandas in one organization. But Master Sivananda could not be persuaded. He had plans. To the first concern, he replied: "Go ahead. I will work through you. Don't worry." And to the second, he said, laughing: "From now on, she will be known as Swami Satchidananda Mataji [mother], and you can use Yogiraj [master of Yoga], the title that I gave you. You will be known as Yogiraj Swami Satchidananda." The matter was settled and the Trincomalee Divine Life Society branch was opened in September 1953.

By 1955, Gurudev's travels and service around the island of Ceylon had increased greatly. Moreover, Trincomalee was located a great distance away from many other parts of Ceylon, so when a group of devotees decided to start a branch of the Divine Life Society in the hill capital of Kandy, they persuaded Gurudev that if he were situated in this centrally located city, it would be easier for him to drive all around Ceylon in order to satisfy the many requests for his presence. Thus, in October of 1955, Gurudev and the Kandy devotees founded a new *ashram* in Kandy.

Near the *ashram*, there was a minimum security prison camp for inmates who had demonstrated good behavior. The Divine Life Society members built a temple for these men and conducted regular prayer meetings. The success of the program was so great that soon Gurudev and the *ashram* members were asked to provide the same service at Kandy's maximum security facility, Bogambura Prison.

At that time, there were only ten or fifteen men in the capital punishment ward of Bogambura Prison and each inmate was locked in his own tiny cell. Only Gurudev and a few others were allowed to enter the cells to speak with prisoners individually. If Gurudev and his volunteers felt that a particular prisoner was trustworthy, they would suggest to the officials that the man be allowed to come out of the cell for their talks. In addition, they would give inmates holy pictures, books and *mantra*s to occupy their minds. And many of the prisoners found comfort and inspiration. In fact, quite a few men completely reformed and were released from prison. One former inmate, for example, turned his farm into an *ashram* and became a great yogi.

Sadly, not all of these prisoners were able to undergo such positive changes. Indeed, one of them was sentenced to be hanged for murder. On the day of this unfortunate man's execution, Gurudev received a call from the prison warden asking him to come to the prison as soon as possible.

"What's wrong?" Gurudev asked.

"This morning, we are going to hang the condemned prisoner," replied the warden, "and his last request is that you should be here when he is hanged. He wants to be able to die seeing your face. If you feel uncomfortable, Swamiji, we will understand. You are free to refuse. I'm simply telling you his request."

Sri Gurudev gave the request some thought before answering; of course, it would be uncomfortable to watch a person hang. Then, he replied, "Who am I to refuse his last wish? Somehow, he feels that this will help him and I would do anything to bring him comfort at the moment of death. Surely God will give me the strength to face it."

At the prison, as soon as he saw Gurudev, the condemned man ran to him, grabbing his hands, crying, begging and praying: "Please, please bless me so that I may get liberated because of this." Gurudev gave his blessings. Then, the guards led the prisoner to a platform; he stood silently, hands folded in prayer, his eyes totally focused on Gurudev as though he were deeply absorbing his holy vibration. Gurudev stood only three or four feet away, praying for the peace of the man's soul. Even after the hood was placed over his head, the prisoner asked, "Is he still there?" "Yes, yes," came the answer. "The swami is still here." The rope was placed around the man's neck. Praying softly for the condemned man, Gurudev turned as the hanging took place.

Needless to say, this anecdote inspired me when I read it in Gurudev's biography, *Swami Satchidananda: Apostle of Peace*, which was published in 1986, the year that I moved to the *ashram*. Little did I know that ten years later I too would be blessed with the opportunity to serve in prison. I say blessed, because serving in prison is, like Yoga itself, life-transforming.

Faith and Fear Don't Go Together

Treat everyone as God. Feel God's presence in everyone. If you see the entire Universe as a divine representation, you will start going out and serving everyone. –Sri Swami Satchidananda

My own prison experience began in the *ashram* dining hall in the fall of 1996. Reading has been my passion since childhood, and my husband, Snehan, perpetually teases me about reading every poster or sign that enters my field of vision. So, it wasn't surprising that after lunch one day, I noticed a little note posted on the bulletin board in the dining hall. It turned out to be a request for literacy volunteers sent by the principal of the educational program of a nearby prison. With post-graduate degrees in English and English Education, and experience in teaching remedial reading and writing to college students, I knew that my training and experience would be useful. Also, I felt that this would be a great opportunity to serve in the larger community of Buckingham County, the county in central Virginia where Yogaville is located. Reading the note from the prison, I got the feeling that an invaluable, as well as challenging, experience awaited me. Challenging it was. And it was also one of the most rewarding experiences of my life.

As a whole-time member at Satchidananda Ashram, I worked full time, receiving room, board, all personal necessities and a small allowance. Over the years, I served in many *ashram* areas–the *ashram* school, kitchen, Programs Department, Teacher Training, Guest Services–making use of old skills and acquiring new ones and, more significantly, learning to live harmoniously with a group of people whose backgrounds and spiritual perspectives were, at times, very different from my own. By 1996, I had been serving for several years as editor of the *Integral Yoga Magazine* and manager of the Publications Department. A notable characteristic and one of the many challenges of living and working at an *ashram* is that there are always more tasks than people to perform them. Satchidananda Ashram-Yogaville was, and is, no exception. But I convinced the *ashram* administration that I could fulfill my *ashram* duties and also volunteer once a week at the prison.

So about a week later, after a peaceful fifteen-minute drive through the lush, gentle countryside of rural Buckingham, Virginia, I found myself in the parking lot of the Buckingham Correctional Center, a maximum-security facility that housed about a thousand men. From movies and books, I had an idea of what I might encounter; however, even my overactive imagination failed to prepare me for the scene that I was about to enter. It wasn't just the starkness of the landscape, the grim building complex, the layers upon layers of barbed wire, or the signs warning visitors to beware of ferocious drug-detecting dogs (Where, I wondered?). It was the vibration that I sensed even before getting out of the car, a vibration, a feeling of isolation and despair.

Taking a few very deep breaths, I entered the main building. A guard sitting at a table asked for identification and checked to make sure that my name was on the volunteer list for that day. Then I was asked to walk through an electronic detection gate. On the other side of the gate, a guard was waiting to frisk me with a hand-held device. After surrendering my driver's license, receiving an identification card, and signing in, I was escorted and deposited into a space that was the size of a small elevator. There were two heavy metal doors, one behind and one in front of me. The one behind me clanged shut. Then, a disembodied voice asked me to identify myself, after which the door in front of me opened. I was told to walk into the next control center, where the process was repeated. I can't remember now whether I walked through two or three control centers, but what I do remember is that it seemed surreal, even a bit nightmarish. Doors clanging closed behind me before other heavy metal doors opened in front to let me pass through. The air was suffocating, heavy with the smell of industrial detergent. Finally, there were no more control centers. I had entered an area high above a huge yard that was filled with what seemed like hundreds of men, all walking toward a door. I saw feelings of rage and despair, isolation and alienation reflected in some of the dour faces peering up at me as I walked past a large crowd of inmates who had been let out into the yard to go to the canteen for lunch. I tried to imagine what it must be like to spend most of your life in such a tense and intense environment. It crossed my mind that the guards who had to work there to earn a living were, in a sense, imprisoned, too.

Like most people, I had never been in a prison, and I couldn't stop thinking that it looked just like it did in the movies. Every so often, though, an inner voice kept reminding me that this was the real thing. As I walked along the raised sidewalk at the edge of the yard, some of the inmates smiled and called, "Hi; how're you?" Others screamed, "Hey, who are you? Are you a teacher? Can I come to your class?" They all stared. Some of the guards (armed men and women) offered a friendly hello, but others looked as hard and as intimidating as the inmates. I could feel unseen eyes peering at me from the guard towers that loomed imposingly above the complex. Fear and fascination bubbled up from the depths of my psyche. "Repeat your *mantra*. Repeat your *mantra*," prompted the voice within. I did. I even managed to smile as I waited for someone to open a door that would take me out of the yard area and into another part of the labyrinthine complex.

Finally, a guard led me into the educational wing of the prison and into the office of the school principal, a pleasant, mild-mannered man with whom I felt an instant rapport. When he learned that I had taught college English, he very excitedly explained that he needed a volunteer to teach a college-level fiction-writing class rather than a literacy course. He looked over my *curriculum vita*–doctorate in English Education/Language Arts, M.A. in English and many graduate credits in Creative Arts Education–and immediately offered me the job. I knew that it would be a challenge, because while I'd taken creative writing classes and had written some poetry and fiction, I'd never taught creative writing. But I accepted.

I learned from the principal that the fiction writing class had been part of a college degree program and that the program had been cancelled. Why had it been cancelled? Because the governor of the state, pressured by constituents who felt that we shouldn't be spending taxpayers' money to fund higher education for prisoners, made the decision to eliminate the program. Prisoners were in prison to be punished, not rewarded. Fortunately, the principal had been able to continue this particular class, whose members were committed, enthusiastic and quite talented, because he had been successful in recruiting volunteer teachers. In fact, whenever a teacher left, another volunteer miraculously appeared. Now it was my turn.

I mentioned earlier that I'd felt a rapport with the principal who interviewed me. As it turned out, he too had lived at an *ashram* for a number of years, studying with a spiritual teacher. But what was even more surprising was that, fifteen years before, he and his wife had brought their newborn daughter to Yogaville to be blessed by Gurudev. As the late poet James Merrill once told me when I was a graduate student, "My dear, there are no accidents in the universe."

A week later, I began teaching my creative writing class and my first class in prison.

Before entering the classroom, I started to feel a little nervous. Luckily I remembered, and took, the down-home advice that the late, great singer Bessie Smith once offered a performer who was suffering from stage-fright: "All you need to do is to think of the people out there as just folks." In any case, I walked into a unique situation with some very special folks and quickly encountered a few more surprises.

During our interview, the principal had warned me, several times, to be extremely cautious around the men and never to disclose anything about my personal life. While he didn't disclose any information about specific individuals, he made sure to let me know that I'd be interacting with men who'd been convicted of such crimes as murder, rape, armed robbery, etc. So, you can imagine my surprise when a guard led me into a classroom, walked out and slammed the door shut. Suddenly, I found myself alone with ten curious male inmates, all seated around a table, all staring at me intensely. There was no guard and I had a suspicion that the door was locked. I have to admit, the situation was downright scary.

I looked at the men, thinking, "Wow, I'm locked in a room, alone with a group of criminals. Well, anything might happen and maybe it will!" At the same time, though, my intuition told me that I had nothing to fear. I realized that this was an opportunity to trust my intuition and to let go of some very deep fears. I remembered how Bessie Smith thought of her audience. I told myself that these guys are also, just folks. My perception shifted, and what I saw behind the tough facades, was a group of very vulnerable souls. My heart opened and compassion conquered fear. I didn't intend to throw caution to the wind, but, without a single doubt, I realized that these men and I had something to give to each other.

As we sized each other up, I remembered learning that in India *ashram* residents are called inmates; so, after introducing myself, to break the ice, I announced that I also lived in an institution where residents were known as inmates. I knew that I wasn't supposed to share any personal information, but I figured that no one would ever imagine that there was an *ashram* in the area. Well, my announcement certainly broke the ice, as one of the men casually asked, "Oh, do you live at Yogaville?" Caught off guard, so to speak, I nodded. He continued with great warmth and affection: "What

I love about Swami Satchidananda is that when people ask him if he's a Hindu, he answers that he's an Undo." For a moment, I thought that perhaps my mind was playing tricks on me, that maybe because the environment was so foreign and so intimidating, I was imagining a conversation about things familiar and safe. But the student's laughter was real as he noticed the expression on my face: astonishment.

He went on to explain that he had begun studying Yoga in prison through a correspondence course offered by a swami whose name I was vaguely familiar with. Also, for years, he had been studying Integral Yoga, reading Gurudev's books, which he ordered from the Integral Yoga Distribution Catalog. He even knew some of the ashramites who worked in Distribution, because he communicated with them from time to time. What's more, this man even had a Sanskrit spiritual name, Devdas (servant of God). Devdas told me that many prisoners in the facility joined religious clubs or "communities," whose members—Christian, Muslim, Jewish, Native American, Buddhist, etc.—met one evening a week. He belonged to a group called the Buckingham Monastic Community, which had been founded some years back by a Buddhist inmate. Members of the Buckingham Monastic Community considered themselves to be monks. They meditated regularly, studied scriptures and spiritual books, did *Hatha Yoga* and were committed to celibacy and non-violence. And while they focused on Yoga and Eastern philosophy, they embraced an interfaith approach to spiritual life. You can imagine how curious I was at this point about this "community," and I felt honored when Devdas invited me to attend a Monday evening meeting. Suddenly, the environment didn't seem quite so alien to me. I found myself, in fact, among a group of people who were interested in both writing and Yoga, two interests that had been an integral part of my own life for many years.

Since childhood, I've had a passion for literature. And the students in the fiction-writing class at the prison shared this passion. As a matter of fact, these men were not only avid readers, they were also excellent writers; in fact, some had already published their work. One fellow, who wrote riveting short stories–crime stories!–mentioned that his mom was a published poet and had been the first woman professor emeritus in the Virginia community college system.

All the men were grateful for the writing class, for it gave them an opportunity to refine their writing and to meet regularly with others who had similar interests and talents. And they really appreciated the opportunity to communicate directly with someone who lived and worked outside the prison. That their new instructor was a woman boosted their enthusiasm, because it brought some feminine energy to the all-male maximum security facility.

Although some of the students were a bit shy, they were all friendly, serious about writing and eager to make me feel comfortable. In fact, as the weeks went by, the men became very protective of me, offering some inside information about prison culture so that I had some deeper understanding of their experience.

A few days after the first writing class, I decided to accept the invitation to a Monday evening gathering of the Buckingham Monastic Community. This was the first of many gatherings that I attended.

On that first Monday night, there were about eight men in the group. Devdas jumped up excitedly to greet me. He introduced me to the other men, all of whom welcomed me warmly. During the evening, I learned that awhile back an acquaintance of mine–a former Yogaville resident–had taught accounting in the prison college program and occasionally he had attended Monastic Community meetings, where he led meditation and *Hatha Yoga* sessions. I also discovered that it wasn't only Devdas who had studied Yoga. Apparently, two other men had been studying Yoga, including Integral Yoga, for many years. One of them was Vishnudas. In fact, Vishnudas had been a close disciple of a well-known Indian spiritual teacher. He had been seriously studying *Raja Yoga* (the path of mind control through meditation), *Jnana Yoga* (the path of self-analysis) and *Bhakti Yoga* (the path of devotion) for many years. He was familiar with many Sanskrit mantras, chants and prayers, which he knew by heart, and had been doing vigorous *sadhana*, spiritual practice, regularly for years.

Vishnudas told me that before he was incarcerated, he had been the director of a spiritual retreat center. When I met him, he had been in prison for about thirteen years. During this time, he was diagnosed with a serious medical condition and he'd had two near-death experiences, experiences that compelled him to dedicate his life to spiritual study, especially to the teachings of Yoga and the *Vedas* (ancient Hindu scriptures) and to share what he was learning with other prisoners.

Although Vishnudas did tell me something about his background, I had no desire to know why the men were incarcerated. It's not that I didn't care, but I didn't want to make any *a priori* judgments based on what I'd heard about their past. Rather, I preferred to know these individuals in the present, from my own experience.

For the first several weeks, I felt like a tourist, as though I had entered a strange, exotic culture. And like a tourist, I held certain preconceptions and opinions, surely; but also like a tourist, I felt open and childlike, the way we feel when we're visiting a foreign country for the first time. This prison country had its own language, its own culture and its own values and conventions. I was interacting with people who had journeyed into realms that, perhaps, I could never imagine. Yes, they had sad stories to tell of incredibly dysfunctional families, of drug abuse and alcoholism, of uncontrolled rage and self-hatred. But they also had positive stories to share of heroism in the military—in the Gulf War, for example—of supportive and loving families and friends and of a strong faith in God. Indeed, one story, told by another long-term prison yogi, Mohandas (his Yoga spiritual name) falls into the realm, at least for me, of the mystical, if not the miraculous.

Mohandas was a gentle, soft-spoken man in his early forties. He had read most of Gurudev's books, adored Swami Sivananda and other Yoga masters and had been studying all the branches of Yoga for the past twenty-four years—in prison. Mohandas told me that Yoga had completely changed his life. And this time, curiosity got the better of me. I asked him how he came to practice Yoga in prison and he related the following account.

At the time that he was first incarcerated, he was so aggressive that he had to be placed in solitary confinement. Here, he became even more violent, wild, like a caged animal and he felt particular animosity toward the guard assigned to his cell. He really hated this guard and, before long, he made up his mind to kill him. Mohandas focused all his attention on figuring out a way to harm this guard. After a while, to give his mind a break, he remembered that someone had sent him a book and he picked it up to see what it was about. As it happened, it was a book about Yoga and, somehow, the subject caught his interest. After a few hours of reading, Mohandas fell asleep. When he woke up, he felt different. When he began to think about the guard, he realized that he no longer had an urge to hurt him. What's more, he felt strangely peaceful. Mohandas told me that that feeling of peacefulness never left, even after twenty-four years in prison. Mohandas was one of the most gracious, gentle and relaxed people that I ever met.

Not long after my tenure at the prison was over (I was moving to France and, coincidentally, the prison was put on lock-down, which meant that all volunteer programs were suspended), I received news that Mohandas had been transferred to a minimum security prison. I'll always remember how, at the Monastic Community meetings, Mohandas sat quietly doing *japa* (repetition of a *mantra*) with the *mala* (rosary beads) that never left him. He had become a real yogi. Actually, during those meetings, all the men behaved like yogis. We meditated together, I taught *Hatha Yoga*, we discussed spiritual issues, and we watched videotapes of Gurudev's *satsang*s (spiritual gatherings). In fact, after viewing the first tape, the men asked me to bring one every week. I began to realize that my spiritual community was expanding, and I felt quite at home with my prison *sangha*, my prison spiritual community.

In time, the students in the fiction writing class heard, through the grapevine, about our Monastic Community meetings, and, one by one, nearly all of them joined the Monastic Community. They all seemed to have developed a hunger for spiritual community, for interfaith discussions, and for the yogic teachings and practices. They were genuinely happy whenever I brought them books donated by the *ashram*.

In the Eastern tradition, it is said that when the student is ready, the master appears. Perhaps, this was the case at the Buckingham Correctional Center. At least that's how I perceived it when some of the men asked me whether I thought that Swami Satchidananda might consider coming to visit them. Although Gurudev was already more than 80 years old, he was still traveling, invited to give talks around the US and abroad, and these students lived right in the neighborhood. I suggested that they send him an invitation and they did. As a matter of fact, they wrote the invitation with great care, making sure that it was perfect in every way (one definition of Yoga is: perfection in action). Needless to say, they were overjoyed when Gurudev accepted their invitation and, immediately, they began to plan the event.

The group wanted Gurudev's visit to the prison to mirror Yogaville's Saturday evening *satsang*. I described the typical format and the men organized the whole event. They wrote questions on index cards, they reserved the nicest room, and they put up flyers announcing the program. They even arranged an especially comfortable chair for Gurudev, just the way we did it at the *ashram*. After several changes in schedule (we continually reminded ourselves of Gurudev's practical advice: *Make no appointments and you'll have no dis-appointments*), the long-awaited day, August 5, 1996, finally arrived.

That evening all the students from the fiction writing class came, all the Buckingham Monastic Community members were there, many other inmates attended, and the principal of the prison's education department was there, too. In honor of Gurudev, one inmate read a lovely poem that was set to music. And, just like at our regular *ashram satsang*s, Gurudev was presented with a set of index cards that contained questions for him to answer. (I have included the transcript of that talk at the end of this chapter.)

After the talk, all the men came up to meet Gurudev. I was so happy to be able to introduce my spiritual teacher to this special group of people. Many of the men asked Gurudev for his autograph. Some asked him to sign one of his books, while others had nothing for him to sign but their baseball caps. And they asked him to return. The joy was palpable.

As I mentioned earlier, I am truly grateful to have had the extraordinary opportunity to serve in the prison community, to encounter and interact with kindred spirits whose lives have taken such a different turn from my own, and to experience in such a challenging environment the transformative power of Yoga. When I led the Monastic Community's silent meditation sessions, the sensation of peace was so powerful that it cut right through any fear that I, a woman, had of sitting in a room, the door shut, with a group of male maximum-security convicts. And when I guided the men into deep relaxation, my heart opened wide as I watched each man lying on the floor as peaceful, as serene and as lovable as a sleeping child. Then, there was the party. The men organized a party as a way of thanking me for spending time with them. They brought the healthiest snacks that they could find in the prison canteen, snacks they thought would be appropriate for a yogi, they said; and they even served herbal tea. I was so touched when they asked me to bring a Yogaville meditation and *Hatha Yoga* schedule, so that they could follow it on a daily basis.

Finally, I'll never forget the love, respect and hope that I saw in the eyes of those prisoners who came to listen to Gurudev as he assured them that they could experience freedom, inner freedom, in whatever situation they found themselves, whether inside a prison or out on the street.

Swami Satchidananda at the Buckingham Correction Center
Dillwyn, Virginia, August 5, 1996

Karma

It's hard to come into a correctional institution and say that the inmates are fortunate. But, before I answer your questions, I would like to say that you are, in a way, fortunate people.

Just now, we heard a poem written by a member of the Buckingham Monastic Community. As monastic members, you know the advantage of sitting in meditation and, here, you are fully protected, with food guaranteed, and nobody to bother you. So, you have ample opportunity to meditate. You can think about this opportunity instead of having any negative feelings of: "Why am I here?"

Maybe you didn't even commit a crime; but, still, if you are here as a monastic community, you should know that there is a *karma* theory. That is, if you did something sometime, you have to face it some other time. You might not have done anything this time, but you do believe in reincarnation and pre-incarnation. You might have done something before, in your past lives, but you escaped from that and now you are facing the result of it; now you have to face it. Because, once we do something, we cannot avoid facing the consequences. That's what you call the *karma* theory: *what you sow, you reap*. So, even if you are here and you are innocent, you should not say, "I am being punished unnecessarily." You might have done something in a past life and you are purging it. The Bible says, "Blessed are the sufferers." Why should it say, "Blessed are the sufferers"? Can the sufferers be blessed? The reason is that if we want to wash our *karma*, we have to undergo some suffering.

For example, the *karma* is like dirt in our life. If your clothing gets dirty, what do you do with it? Do you fold it, put it on an altar and pray, "Get cleaned"? No. ["Wash it," someone from the group answers.] Yes, wash it. Washing means that the item undergoes a lot of suffering. You have to immerse it in water, apply soap, rub it, scrub it, and boil it. It's all suffering. But your intention is not to destroy the clothing. You are doing it all just to clean up the dirt. You are interested in the *dhoti*, in the clean cloth. You want to remove the dirt, but it cannot be done without going through the suffering. After washing, there will still be some wrinkles. How do you straighten them out? With a hot iron. That's also another part of suffering. "Blessed are the sufferers" means that by the suffering, we are cleaning our past *karmas*, whatever we have done in this birth or in the previous birth.

Before I go further, do you believe in rebirth or pre-birth? Does anybody have any doubt? We lived before. Do you know that? [Some group members answer: "I'm not sure" and "I have mixed feelings."] Mixed feelings. Okay. Then I have to discuss that first.

Let's say that this birth is the only birth for us, that we neither lived before, nor will we live afterward. But you do believe that God created people? Is that so?

Inmate: "Yes."

Gurudev: "God created everybody. Is God impartial or partial?"

Inmate: "Impartial."

Gurudev: "Impartial."

Inmate: "I'm not sure about that either, but I'll say impartial."

Gurudev: "You'll say impartial. If an impartial God were to create people for the first time, why should He create them with so many differences? Some in poor families, some in rich families. Some handicapped, some in good health. Some knowledgeable, some dull-headed. Does God take a fancy in creating like that? You don't have an answer for that. The only answer is that we sowed the seed before and, in this birth, we are facing what we sowed before. We have to believe in reincarnation in order to understand the changes, the recurrences in upbringing and the differences in life status.

Question: Then why do we not recall past lives clearly? Are we destined to live a life and, then, just to throw it away without remembering it?

Sri Gurudev: Well, we can recall if we want. But can you recall exactly what you did a year before on this day, at this time?

Question: If it were important to me, yes.

Sri Gurudev: Okay. If it were important, you could recall that, also. You can go back. It's a chain. It's not forgotten. It's all recorded in our minds. For example, Lord Buddha meditated, and he envisioned ten past lives. It's possible, but we don't have to spend time on that. Why? There's no point in knowing why this is happening. Instead, we should think, "This has happened. There must be a good reason. I did something. I don't know what, why, how, but it happened here. How can I avoid it? How can I root it out? There's no point in thinking of the past. Think of the present: "What can we do now to take care of our past mistakes?"

So, that is what you call *karma*. *Karma* means that when you do an act, you face a result. The Sanskrit word *karma* is used for both the present act and its result. Both are called *karma*. You might have done something in the past, so you are facing this situation here. Okay, accept it and take it as a sort of cleaning process: "I am being helped to clean my past *karma*." That is what is called *tapasya* in Patanjali's *Yoga Sutras*. *Tapasya* means to heat, to boil, to burn. You are burning your own sins, mistakes committed in the past or in the present. And with *tapasya*, by burning it out, you are cleaning it out. Everyone goes through the suffering. Not only those in prison, but even in the outside world. People undergo a lot of suffering, because that is the only way to clean up their past *karmas*. So, instead of having negative feelings–"Oh, he must be the cause for my being here" or "He did something wrong. He told a falsehood. That's why I am here;"–instead of blaming all those people, accept that what has happened has happened; but don't blame others. Blame your own past *karma*. And then, ask, "What can I do now? The answer should be: "Let me clean out my *karma*."

No Pain, No Gain

Don't think of others as enemies. It's not somebody else who can do something to you. Even if anybody wants to do something, he cannot. In fact, there is a theory: nothing happens to you if you do not deserve it. Nobody can help you or hinder you. Nobody can make you happy or make you unhappy if you do not deserve it. The others are only instruments. If you deserve it, you face it; there's no point in blaming somebody else for that. If you keep on blaming others, you are never going to find out why you are in the situation. So, this opportunity is given to you by God to clean up your past *karma*. Think, "Let me get cleaned." That way, you can accept pain. It's painful only when you don't want to accept the pain. When you accept the pain, when you understand the pain, you will, in a way, enjoy it.

For example, two ladies who don't know each other come to a clinic. One woman goes to the doctor, complaining, "I have a stomachache. Could you give me some medicine?" The doctor gives her some medicine and she goes out. Another woman goes in, "Doctor,

I should have had my stomachache, the pain, yesterday, but I didn't get it. Can you induce some pain?" Who could that be, the woman who goes to ask the doctor to induce pain? Do you know why she might ask? Is she crazy? Can you find out the reason for it? She says, "According to my doctor, I should have had the pain yesterday and I didn't have it; so could you induce the pain?" What for? She was expecting a baby! You get it? She's asking for pain, because she expects a gain. Without the pain, she won't have the gain.

Another example: You go to the doctor to have an operation. You pay the money, the doctor's fees, and you get the operation, which is a painful thing. Why do you want to do that? Because you know the gain of it, right? The pain that comes to us if we understand it and accept it is no more pain at all. It may be superficially painful but, within, it's a joyful thing.

Going back to the previous example, when the doctor introduced the pain to the woman, the woman was happy. Why? "I am going to have a baby now." Do you understand that? That's what. Pain should be understood properly. If you understand it, if it comes—and we don't have to go looking for it or take it by force—accept it. You may not know the reason, but think, "Well, I must have done something, and the pain is going to clean me up. I am going to become a better person. So, let me have that." It is in that sense that one of the Beatitudes says, "Blessed are the sufferers." Having said that, let me go to your questions.

The Supernatural

Question: How do you explain the supernatural, such as supernatural activities or supernatural beings—the unexplained and unseen?

Sri Gurudev: We call something supernatural because it's not natural for us. In our limited understanding, within our time and space, it's not natural. But supernatural is natural in a different realm. So it's always there, but we don't see it. We see only within a limited space. For example, this is plain water for me. But take a drop and see the drop under an electronic microscope. What do you see? Do you see water there? You see millions of animals. Yet, it looks like an innocent drop of water. That is supernatural.

Why? Because it is beyond our understanding. If we expand our understanding to that level, then it's no longer supernatural. That's why we say about supernatural things "Oh, it is extraordinary. You cannot do that." But somebody can do it. Thus, all those supernatural activities are based on expansion of the mind.

Your mind functions only within a limited area. But you can expand the mind. You can go into the unconscious, the subconscious and the superconscious. Mind stays in different levels. Normally, we act or function on the conscious level. When we go to sleep, in deep sleep it is on the unconscious level. When we dream, it is subconscious. But–more than the conscious, subconscious, and unconscious levels–there is a fourth dimension called the *superconscious*. It's all in the mind. So, those who develop their mental capacities can do supernatural things. But, still, it's all in the mental realm. Total liberation comes when you go beyond the mind.

Sometimes supernatural activities are called *siddhis*. Psychic powers are called *siddhis* in Sanskrit. For instance, some people can read minds; others can pass through walls or walk on water. These are all supernatural powers, accomplishments. *Siddhi* can be translated as "accomplishment." When you pray, when you meditate deeply, when you have gained some mastery over your mind, the mind gets more powerful; the mind can do many things that you normally cannot do. But those *siddhis* are also, in a way, a hindrance to us, because we want to rise above the mind and see the Self, or the soul clearly. But when people acquire supernatural powers, they get egoistic: "Oh, I can do this!" And that ego creates a big block. So, sometimes, when you have deep meditation, supernatural powers come automatically. Naturally, they will come. However, sensible people avoid and go beyond that. Sensible people won't get caught in that, because it's the ego's net.

Focus the Mind

Question: Can I do other meditations along with japa *[repetition of a mantra]?*

Sri Gurudev: You can. But the point of meditating is to focus the mind on one point. Concentration means that when the mind runs here and there, you bring it back to the point of meditation and you perfect the concentration; then, it becomes meditation. This means that the mind should stay focused on one point. If you are going to have different types of meditation, the mind runs to various places, various objects. So, whichever method is good, select one. Even though all meditations are equally good, you have to select one that is pleasant to you, one that suits your temperament and your taste and, then, stick to that. Otherwise, if you practice different meditations, it's almost like digging wells in too many places. Wherever you dig, you will get water. But by the time you dig ten feet, if somebody says, "No, no, no, that's not the right place; dig here," you go there and dig fifteen feet. Then, another person comes: "That's not the right place; go to another place." So, if you keep on digging shallow wells in different places, you'll never get water, but you have put so much effort into the project already. If you had put all the effort in one place, you would have gotten water sooner.

That's why we have different types of meditations. Even though all are equally good, stay with one practice. The simplest practice is *japa*. The mind has to be engaged in one thing. Here you are giving it a *mantra*, or a small prayer–not too long, not too big. And then, you keep repeating it. *Japa* means to repeat the same thing, and the mind dwells in that. When the mind is fully focused on the *mantra*, it forgets all other thoughts. Then, if you are deeply involved in it (which is what we call meditation), at one point, even that will slip away, because even all these meditations are like catalytic agents.

Do you know what a catalytic agent is? It's a counteracting agent. Take, for example, soap. Soap is a catalytic agent. Why? Why do you use soap? To remove the dirt from the cloth, right? In order to remove the dirt from the cloth, you buy a little soap. I call that soap another form of dirt, though it is nicely named, nicely scented, like Lux or Ivory. Beautifully named, yes, but also dirt, because only dirt can remove other dirt. So, you add on new dirt and rub it in well. Do you know what happens at that time? When you add new dirt to the cloth, the old dirt sees new dirt coming and gathers there to greet the new dirt: "Hello. Who are you? You seem to be good smelling. What's your name? You seem to have a nice name."

Dirts of the same feather flock together, no? So, the old and new dirt try to chum up. And the laundryman knows the right time. When they all forget the cloth and chum up, he dips the cloth in the water and then takes it out. What happens? The old dirt stays in the water. But do you want to have the new dirt in the cloth? No. Even that has to go. That has finished its job. That's what you call a catalytic agent.

Thus, even *japa* meditation, all your practices are catalytic agents. Stick to one thing until you clean up your mind. Then, even that is gone. You are totally free. That's what you call *nirvana*. Lord Buddha calls it *nirvana*. *Nirvana* means total nakedness, nothing to cover or color. So stay with one practice and keep doing it until your mind becomes totally, totally focused and absorbed in that practice. That is called *samadhi*.

You know, in his *Yoga Sutras*, Patanjali talks about that *samadhi*. *Samadhi* means that your mind comes to a well-balanced state. *Samaha* means "equanimity," "balance." The mind is pure. No changes in the mind. No fluctuations in the mind. And that is what is meant by, "Blessed are the pure in heart." That's one of the Beatitudes: "Blessed are the pure in heart." What happens then? "They shall see God." In that pure heart, in that unshakeable, steady mind, you can experience the God within you. In fact, it is for this experience that all the practices are performed. But each individual selects a practice according to his or her taste and temperament. That's why, as you mentioned, when people ask me, "Do you believe in Hinduism?" I reply that I believe in *Undoism*, because religions are all different catalytic agents. You can use Catholic soap, Protestant soap, Hindu soap, Muslim soap, Jewish soap. It doesn't matter. Whatever soap I use, all I want is my mind to be clean.

However, if you don't realize that and if you don't accept that, you say, "Oh, this is the only way or that is the only way," and you fight with each other. In fact, the whole world is in turmoil because human beings fight in the name of God and religion. But the prophets who gave us God and religion, where are they? Jesus, Moses, Buddha, Muhammad, they are all up in heaven. And if you happen to go there, you will see them playing together, sitting and playing cards. They don't have qualms, quarrels among themselves. They are all happy together. You go up and see. Maybe you can ask Christ, "Sir, they're asking you to come back. When is the Second Coming?" And Christ will answer, "No, no, no, no. Don't call me. I've had enough. In our name, see what is happening down there. We don't want to get involved in that."

That's why it's time for us to accept various approaches. There need not be only one way. Once, I was in the Vatican, waiting to have an audience with the Pope. Some of the Cardinals were there. One of the Cardinals who knew about my work casually asked me, "Swami, what do you mean by 'truth is one, paths are many?' You put all the various religions together and accept all that. How can there be so many paths to one truth?" I said, "Sir, I am not here to explain the Bible to you. You know it better than I do. But I would like to ask you one question: Where is the city of Vatican? "Oh, it's in Rome." "Well, have you heard the saying, 'All roads lead to Rome'? When your little Rome can have so many roads, why cannot our home up there have a few more extra roads?"

That is to say, whatever road you choose to take, it doesn't matter. To make another analogy, all the rivers, even though they have separate names, separate colors, separate tastes, they all fall into the sea. All the waters fall into the sea. And once they fall into the sea, do they still have their names? The Missouri, the Mississippi, the Amazon, and the Ganges in India, they all fall into the same sea, and you don't separate them. They all have the name *holy sea*. You see? When you see that, you cannot say, "Mine is the only river that can fall into this ocean." Take your own river; follow that one; let others take and follow their rivers; and then, know that we will all fall into the same ocean. There's no need to fight in the name of race, religion, God.

Good and Evil

Question: What is evil?

Sri Gurudev: That's a good question. If God created everything, God would have created evil, also. Do you agree that God created everything? (Inmates: "Yes.") So then, who created evil? (Inmates:

"God.") God created evil. Why? God has both good and evil, and God wants you to choose whichever you like and tells you, "Better to choose good; don't follow evil." But if you decide to follow evil, God allows you to go through that and face the consequences and then, learn from that and come back to good.

Positive and negative, both are equally important. The light burns. Can it burn only with the positive wire? It needs the negative wire, also. So, good and evil are both needed for us to use our intelligence. When God created Adam, what did God say? The first thing was, "Adam, don't eat the apple or the fruit," right? God said, "Don't eat the fruit." But when Adam reached for the fruit, where was God? God could have said, "Adam, stop it!" But God didn't. Why? God gave Adam good advice and Adam disobeyed. God allowed Adam to disobey. Why? Because only by disobeying and by facing the consequences does one turn to the right. So, evil is necessary to give you experience, bad experience, so that you can turn to good. That's why the world is a mixture of good and evil and that's why evil is equally important.

Another example: What is something evil? The hair on the head is good. It gets all the nice shampoo and scent and this and that as long as it is on the head. But suppose one hair falls onto the dinner plate. You shampooed the hair and you adored it when it was on your head. Now, the same hair is on the dinner plate, but you don't adore it there. This means that a right thing in the wrong place is evil. That is to say, it depends upon how you use that object. In one sense, there's nothing evil, nothing good. Everything is neutral. That's why we call it "nature." Nature is neutral.

Take a pen knife, for example. Is it good or bad? Fire: good or bad? Poison: good or bad? Deadly cobra poison can be a medicine. If you know how to use something, it's good. If you don't know how to use it, it's bad. If you cut the fruit with a knife, a knife is good. But if you cut the throat? So, who makes the knife good or bad? You do. If you know how to use it, there's nothing bad in this world. To give a further example: a stone. Is it good or bad? If you throw it at somebody, it's bad. If you build a house, it's good. Take anything in life. Take selfishness. Selfishness is, in a way, also good. Why?

Because selfishness teaches you a lesson: not to be selfish. Because by selfishness, you get into trouble and then you learn a lesson.

God didn't create anything without any use. Sometimes people say, "Oh, I don't know what I am doing here. I am really a good-for-nothing person. I'm not useful to anybody. I am not doing anything." I tell that person, "No; you have a use. You know what use? You are an example for others not to be like you, right?" We have to have an example, no? So, that is a use for evil.

Christhood

Question: Do you believe in Jesus Christ? Do you believe that Jesus Christ was a real person who walked on the earth; and, if so, do you believe that he was the Son of God who became flesh to save man?

Sri Gurudev: I do believe in Jesus Christ. But Christ is not a man. Christ is an attainment–Christhood expressed in that body which you call Jesus Christ. Like Buddha. Buddha is not a person. It's Buddhahood, *Bodhisattva*. A totally enlightened being is called Buddha. That was expressed through a person. You call him Buddha. Otherwise, how can you say, "May Jesus Christ be born in you?" If Christ is a person, how can he be born in you? It's an experience. And that experience was expressed to us, lived among us, through a body, as a human body that we call Jesus Christ. But, now, the body is no more. Can you say that Jesus Christ is not there? Experience is always there. These bodies and the symbols are vehicles to express certain qualities. In this way, I believe that Jesus Christ was alive and that, as a human being, he walked on the earth and that he was the Son of God. But the only thing I don't want to say is that he was the *only* Son of God. Why? God created you and me, right? If God created everything and everybody, then are we not children of God? Then how can Jesus have claimed, "Only I am the Son of God?" No. We adore Jesus, respect him. And because of that we say to him, "Oh, you are the only Son." But that doesn't mean that you are not that, also. We are all children of God and we can have, equally, the same experience, but Jesus brought it out. That is, we can express the same Christhood, Buddhahood, Muhammadhood. The experience is the same.

However, because this experience is manifested through particular individuals, we call them experienced people, and we adore them and respect them. But that experience belongs to every one of us, because God made everybody in God's own image. We are all God's image. It is there in us. We have to realize that. That's what you call *God-realization*. How do we realize that we are God? "Blessed are the pure in heart. They shall see God in them."

Thus, what we call spiritual practices serve to clean up the mind, calm the mind, steady the mind like a mirror. The mind becomes a mirror. In that mirror you see yourself as God. If the mirror is unclean, you see your image as unclean. So, clean up the mirror.

Now, I will ask you another question. Do you all have faces? Does everyone have a face? Yes? Are you sure? How do you know that you have a face? Have you seen it? How did you see it? Did you see your face? Oh, you say that you have seen your face in the mirror. But what you've seen in the mirror is not your face. In the mirror, you've seen a reflection of your face, but you have not seen *your* face (even though you do have a face). Because, since you are the subject, you can never become an object of yourself. That is, you can see only the reflection. Likewise, you are God. If you want to see yourself as God, you can see only a reflection of you. But God reflects where? In a clean mirror. For instance, you see your face in a mirror. Suppose the mirror is crooked. How would you see your face? Crooked. Do you run to the hospital? No. You correct the mirror, right?

In the same way, when you think that you are not clean, that you are this or that, it's not true. You are the pure Self, the image of God. You are seeing your image in a dirty mirror, which is your mind. The color of the mind shows that you are a colored person. But *you* are not colored. Your mind is colored. Your mind is crooked. You see, you are not crooked. Your reflector is crooked. The reflector is the mind. Clean up the mind. That's why I refer to the Beatitude, to which I would like to add a few more words: "Blessed are the pure in heart. They shall see themselves as God." Because you are the image of God. How do you know that you are the image of God? You have to see it. How do you see it? You have to have a mirror. What's your mirror? The mind. So, clean up the mind and you see yourself as God.

A Good Shave

Question: Consider the barber who shaves all the people who live in a village and who do not shave themselves. Does the barber shave himself?

Sri Gurudev: Who asked this question? You are the poet. Unfortunately, the barber cannot give a good shave if he doesn't know how to shave himself. He has to know how to shave himself. If he doesn't know how to shave himself, he can't do the best job. So, it comes from within. You can give somebody what you have; you cannot give somebody what you do not have. So first, the barber has to learn how to shave himself better. Then, he will have a good shave, a clean shave. But, unfortunately, we are all trying to shave others. That's what the world is going through. We want transformation outside. You want everybody to change, but you don't want to change yourself. However, if you don't change yourself, you cannot see a clean person outside, because you see the whole world through your eyes. If your eyes are jaundiced, you will see everybody wearing yellow. Correct your eyes and you will see clearly.

Self-reformation is more important than changing others, but we are always trying to change others, not ourselves. So, to go back to the analogy, the barber has to shave himself well in order to give a good shave outside, because the world is created by our own mind. What we think, we see outside. For example, a crook will always see everyone as a crook. He won't see a really good person. And a good person will always see some good in everybody, because he sees people with his own good heart, with good eyes. The other fellow doesn't see that because his eyes are bad. That's why, all the lessons, all the lessons in every scripture, ultimately, come down to this saying: *Know yourself.* You should know yourself, who you are, first; and, then, you have known others. Otherwise, you are projecting your image onto others. The world is a clean place.

To make another analogy, we have seen movies, right? How does the movie house function? What is there on the screen before the movie starts? The screen is clear, all white, is it not so? A crystal clear, silver screen. There's nothing wrong with the screen. Then, go to the projection room, where the image is projected. Behind the film, there is clear light, correct? The projection room has clear light inside it. Outside, there is a clear screen. How do the pictures come? In between the film rolls. There's nothing wrong with the original light or the outside screen. It all depends upon the film roll.

Our mind is like that. Our mind is a film roll. We register so many things. We record so many things with colors and no colors. Our Self is the light. The image of God is the light. The world is the screen. You project onto the screen, onto the world, what you have recorded here in the mind. Clean up your mind and you see a clean world. So, it all boils down to one thing: clean up your mind, clean up your mind, clean up your mind!

Loss of Faith

Question: What can be done for a friend who loses his faith and abandons his belief in all things intangible?

Sri Gurudev: Ask him how he knew who his father was. I ask you: How do you know your father? Yes, your mother told you. But your mother could have pointed to anybody, so that means that you believed your mother's words. Even to know your father, you have to believe in somebody's words, in your mother's words. So start with that particular belief and work with it; and if your father behaves like a father, your belief enhances, it develops. But we have to have at least a little faith to start working, even if you believe only in yourself.

Once, I was in Moscow, talking to some monks there, Russian Orthodox monks. But I didn't know Russian and the monks didn't know English, so I had to use an interpreter. The government gave me an interpreter, a Communist woman who interpreted our talks. And when monks sit together and talk, what do they talk about? God, God, God. Too many times "God." And this woman got tired of translating "God." At one point, she looked at me and said, "We are non-believers!" And I asked her, "My child, all right; you cannot believe. But, tell me, what is it that you don't believe?" "Oh, I don't believe in the church. I don't believe in the Bible. I don't believe in all these rituals." "Okay," I replied. "You don't have to. But do you believe in friendship? Do you have friends?" "Yes," she answered. "So, you believe in friendship. Do you believe in love? You are a beautiful person." "Yes," she said. Then, I went one step further. "Do you believe in comradeship? (You know, Russians call each other 'comrade.') Do you believe?" "YES!" She sat up, "YES!" She was a staunch communist. "You said that you are a non-believer," I told her. "Yet, you seem to believe in so many things. How can you call yourself a non-believer?" "I guess I'm not," she replied. And I said, "Remember that what you believe in is real religion: friendship, universal brotherhood, love, camaraderie. Those qualities are what really make a person religious, not just going to church and reading the Bible. If a person doesn't believe in these things, what good is it to go to the Bible? Religions are there to teach you how to believe in friendship, universal brotherhood, universal love. So, in that sense, I would say that you are the real religious person." The woman thought, "Huh?" And she thoroughly changed. In fact, when we left for Leningrad, she came to the railway station to see us off and with tears in her eyes, she said, "I wish I could come with you all."

We all have beliefs. Maybe you don't have to believe what someone else believes, but you have your own belief. Start with that. The other thing is that life, itself, will teach you to believe in something. Why? Because with life everything is an obstacle. For example, say you believe in money. Do you think that money will make you happy always? Are all rich people happy? Are all the powerful kings happy? We have seen in our time, for instance, the Shah of Iran. He was the king of kings. And what happened to him? Toward the end of his life, he didn't even have a country in which he could lie down and rest. And what about Marcos, the late dictator of the Philippines? His wife had 2,000 pairs of shoes. Where is she now? Where is he? So, money is not making people happy. Power isn't making them happy either. The moment you get power, you have to shield yourself in a bulletproof car. I'd rather be an ordinary man than ride in a bulletproof car with too many people to guard me with guns. That person is not happy. No.

Nothing can make you happy. Look at the Olympics. Some people showed their gold medals. You know how many others cried and went away? Some people's happiness made so many other people unhappy. And how long will their happiness last? Until next year, when another person jumps half an inch more? And what about this year's beauty queen who was crowned Queen of the Year? Next year, where is she? She's gone. Or even in this same year, the next day, if she gets a simple pimple, gone is her beauty.

So tell me anything, one thing that will, ultimately, always make you happy. Money doesn't make you happy. Power doesn't make you happy. Position doesn't make you happy. Why? Because you are all depending on other things to be happy. You cannot depend on things to make you happy. That's borrowed happiness. You are happy without anything. Independently, you are happy. Nobody can make you unhappy if you decide not to be unhappy. Nobody. Because *you are happiness personified.* That is the image of God in you. Thus, knowing oneself truly, realizing the Self, is the only way to be always happy. On the other hand, when you don't have faith in that and if you believe in all these things—money, power, position—then experience them. Wherever you go, things will make you happy for awhile; and, then, the same things will make you unhappy. I have seen hundreds of people who won huge amounts of money in the lottery. The very next day, thousands of people came to their door: "I am your friend. I am your cousin," and the income tax officer took half the money away. Ultimately, they were all unhappy.

The purpose of the world is to teach you that nothing is going to make you happy. When you learn enough lessons in the world, then there's no other way for you other than to go back within yourself. That is the reason the world is created. Wherever you turn, temporarily, something or someone will make you happy. But before that, you were unhappy. Temporarily, you are happy. Afterwards, you are unhappy. The world is there to teach us: Don't come to me for happiness, because it is within you. You should learn to be independently happy, not dependently happy. So, tell this gentleman that if he doesn't want to believe in anything, it doesn't matter. Tell him to plunge deeply into the world. Let him get bitten by that. And then one day he will, himself, come back and say, "I am sick of all these things." Don't we hear people saying, "I am sick and tired of the whole thing"? I say that when you are a *sick* person, then you are ready to *seek*, then you become a good *seeker*. Who will be a good *seeker*? The one who becomes a good *sicker* in the world, because you can't force people; you can't make them believe. They have to learn by themselves. When everything fails, they begin to believe in themselves.

The Soul Never Dies

Question: How might I become convinced of the immortality of the individual human soul?

Sri Gurudev: After ten years, you go to a village and you ask for a friend whom you knew and someone says, "Oh, Mr. Albert? He is dead and gone." What does she mean by that? Don't we hear that term, "He or she is dead and gone?" What does it mean, "He is dead and gone?" Gone where? *She is dead and gone.* What is *dead* and what is *gone*?

In today's usage, we use that expression without knowing the meaning. The soul never dies. Never. Because it is the image of God. If God dies, the soul will die. So what dies, then? The body. Actually, the body is not dead completely. It disintegrates. It's composed of materials, elements. That's why the priest, toward the end of the funeral ceremony, what does he say? "Earth to earth, water to water, fire to fire." That means that the elements go back to their elements. The elements made the body and the body disintegrated. But the soul goes off looking for another body, because it still has to enjoy some experiences in life. That's why we are all in this body. Our soul wanted to enjoy something that could be done only as a human, so we got human bodies. But when we finish enjoyment in the human body, suppose we want to enjoy something different, like flying? Can you do it in the human body? No. But your wish should be fulfilled, no? How can it be fulfilled? By giving you a bird's body.

Yes, our wishes, our desires bring bodies to us. We create the body according to our desire. You see somebody and say, "Look at him; he's a crook." He is a good-looking, handsome man, so why do you say that he's a crook? What do you see? The body or the mind? [Someone in the audience says: "You see the actions."] Even without seeing the actions, sometimes you simply say, "Oh, I don't like to see him, his horrible face." Why? The mind is horrible. You are expressing your own inner mind through your face, through your body. You change the mind and thinking, you change the face. Somebody will say, "Oh, he seems to be so happy today." Is she seeing the happiness? What is she seeing? The face. Why? The happiness makes the face look happy. The sadness makes the face sad. That means that every thought makes a change in the body. *As you think, so you become.* Think of good thoughts, you are a good person. Think of sad thoughts, evil thoughts, hateful thoughts, you will become that.

That is what. Our soul carries that thought. Our soul doesn't die. It takes bodies according to its wishes. For instance, sometimes, you think, "Oh, look at him. He is cunning like a fox." He's not a fox; he's a man, yet you call him a fox. But the mind is foxy. That's why, again, all religion is asking us is to take care of the mind, to keep the mind clean, to free the mind from all these dirty thoughts and to let it become a mirror, a clean mirror, so that you can see yourself clean.

Logic and Universal Truth

Question: I am a student of logic, mathematics, physics, that type of thing, and I would call that truth, universal truth. But paradox refers to something that can either be or not be. How do you resolve that?

Sri Gurudev: That's what you call *maya*. In the Hindu tradition, it's called *maya*: that which is not is *maya*, paradox, like the footprints of a bird in the sky. Can the bird leave footprints in the sky? No. But you refer to the "footprints of a bird." It's a paradox. Life, itself, is a paradox. We are all, all of us, wonderful liars. We are all liars. What's your name?

Inmate: "Greg."

Gurudev: "Greg. Since when?

Inmate: "Since I was born."

Gurudev: "And before that?"

Inmate: "I didn't have a name."

Gurudev: "So, it's a temporary name, right? Greg is not your name. Your parents argued between themselves and gave you the name. But before that, you were nothing but an "it." When you were in your mother's womb, everybody pointed at your mother's tummy and what did they ask? "Honey, what is *it* going to be?" That was your name: it. And not only *your* name, but everybody's name. When each of us was in the womb, that was our name, too: it. Do you agree with me?

Greg: "Yes!"

So, we are all *it*. But because there are millions of *its* to distinguish between—this *it* and that *it*—we give different names. And only when the nurse came out of the delivery room and told people, "It's a boy," did you, then, become a boy. *It* is a boy.

Why? Because God is a big *It*. And we are the image of God. We are all *it*. Not just us, but everything. *It* is a microphone. *It* is a cup. *It* is a tape recorder—*it* is, *it* is, *it* is. Is *it* not so? Why do you add an *it* to that? Focus on that point. *It* is a fan. *It* is a roof. *It* is a floor. Originally, *it* is all *it*. Then, *it* got the name and form as floor, roof, microphone and things like that. Thus, universally, we are all *it*.

Probably, you don't like the term *it*. Then *I*. Call yourself *I*. If I ask you, "Please write on the chalkboard who you are, you will write, "I am so-and-so"; "I am a boy"; "I am a girl"; "I am a man"; "I am an officer"; "I am a prisoner." It doesn't matter. I am a doctor. I am a graduate. I am a foolish fellow. I am American. I am Italian. Different answers. I am fat. I am thin. I am sick. I am poor. I am rich. Write down all the answers. What is the common element in all of them? *I am.* So, we all have something in common. What is it? *I am.* All the other things are different. Therefore, which is the better half of the answer? *I am.* Why do we call ourselves, "I am, I am, I am, I am?" Because we are all the image of God. Who is God? God is *I AM*.

Do you know the story of when Moses went to the mountain and God spoke to him? God spoke to Moses and Moses wanted to know who was speaking to him. So Moses asked, "Sir, who is it speaking to me?" And what was God's answer? God said, "I AM." Moses waited for a little while. Nothing more came, so he asked, "Sir, I AM who?" Then only did God say, "Moses, I AM That I AM. I have not become somebody. I have not become a boy or a girl or rich or poor, sick or healthy, American or European. No. I AM." That's why we, even today, call ourselves "I am." That's the image of God in us. But for various reasons—just to play different parts in the drama—we put on different makeup. It has to be different; otherwise, we cannot play. If everybody were to be I AM, then you wouldn't be able to play your part.

You know the chessboard? The board is made of wood and the pawns are made of wood. Yes. They are all nothing but chips of the same block. But when they are carved into King, Queen, Bishop and Pawn and put on the board, they seem to come to life. The Queen wants to go everywhere. Queens have the right to go everywhere, hmm? Even the King has restrictions. In any case, as long as they are on the board, they follow the rules; they have certain names, certain forms, certain duties, certain rights. However, when the game is over, you put them all in a box. Would the Queen refuse to rub against the Bishop there? No, because there is no Queen and no Bishop; they are all chips of the same block. Likewise, we play our part, whatever is given to us, as long as we are on the chessboard of the world, until we are put in the box. And in that box, we don't complain, "Who is next to me?"

So, this is the whole drama going on in the world. In the drama, let us play our parts. Everybody is equally important. Just look at this institution itself. Who is important? Only the officers? Without you fellows, what would be the good of the officers? They would lose their jobs. Therefore, who is important here? ["We are!"] That's what. You keep them in jobs. And we play our games. As long as we play, let us play well, but without forgetting that we are only playing our parts. These are all temporary roles. When this part is over, the costume is taken off. Then, we may have to play another part. It doesn't matter. Otherwise, we are all equal. There's no rich and poor, good and bad. Everybody is equal to play the drama. Thus, accept your part. Play it well until the time comes when you are put in the box. Don't allow your mind to become sad or depressed. No. It's all a drama: "I'm joyful. I'm happy. I'm playing my part." Yes, because you can make yourself happy. Nobody is going to make you happy. Nobody can make you happy. Whatever the condition is, don't forget that. You are the image of God, so you are always happy. This is only temporary. This part will come and go.

Thank you and God bless you all.

Gurudev's talk at the Buckingham Correctional Center in 1996 was his last prison talk. In the following chapters, we'll take a look at how, when and where Gurudev began his service in American prisons.

Chapter 2
A New World

Freedom is what you do with what's been done to you. –*Jean-Paul Sartre*

Even today, almost 40 years after one of America's most well-known music festivals was held in Woodstock, New York, those of a certain age remember the Woodstock Swami.

The legendary Woodstock Festival-Aquarian Exposition–three days of free music, free food and free entertainment (and, as we used to call it, free love)–took place during the summer of 1969 in Max Yasgur's cow pasture. Promoters had expected a few thousand people. They weren't prepared for the 400,000 young people who camped out in the miles of tents. What a sight! And what an experience of flower power it turned out to be!

First, the sun burned intensely. Then, the rain poured down. Not surprisingly, the people in charge were concerned that under these conditions and with so many freedom-loving young people, there might be trouble. What to do? One of the organizers of the festival came up with a unique solution: Swami Satchidananda. Apparently, he had met Gurudev and felt that his peaceful, relaxed manner could have a calming effect on the crowd. So they called. And he came. And, he must have made quite an impression, because he arrived like an angel, floating down from the sky–*literally.*

What happened was that the roads leading up to the site were so choked with cars that Gurudev's car couldn't get through, so he was driven in a police car; but even the police car couldn't get through, so a special helicopter arrived to lift him over the traffic and above the thousands who were milling around. His opening words were:

"My beloved sisters and brothers, I am overwhelmed with joy to see the youth of America gathered here in the name of the fine art of music. In fact, through music we can work wonders... One thing I very much wish you all to remember: with sound we can make or break. On certain battlefields animal sounds are used. Without such sounds–war cries–human beings couldn't become the kind of animals that kill their own brethren. So, I am very happy to see that we are all gathered to create some 'making' sounds rather than 'breaking' sounds to find that peace and joy through the celestial music. I am honored for having been given the opportunity of opening this great, great music festival."

No doubt, Gurudev's encouraging expression of faith in the flower children and his prayers for the success and peace of the celebration helped to insure the harmony that pervaded all three days of the festival.

By the time of Woodstock, the first Integral Yoga Institute, actually an apartment at 500 West End Avenue, on New York's Upper West Side, had been functioning for about three years. Many, if not most, of the young people who implored Gurudev to remain in New York and who organized the center were pot-smokers and drug-users, who thought nothing of arriving to one of Gurudev's lectures high on marijuana or tripping on LSD and blowing cigarette smoke in his face. In fact, some adults who were members of established Yoga centers and Vedanta societies warned him that his reputation would be tarnished if he continued to associate with these uncouth flower children. They couldn't tolerate the "hippies" and didn't want to be around Gurudev if he continued to allow himself to be surrounded by such "pigs." His response was: "I am sorry to hear you say all this. All I can see are their beautiful, searching hearts. What you call pigs are my kids." Gurudev knew that his students' negative habits would drop away in time. He knew that, despite their unconventional appearance, they were sincere. And it wasn't too long before many of the young people gave up drugs, smoking, and drinking and learned to be clean and neat. Also, a number of them asked to be trained to be *Hatha Yoga* teachers. The hippies were becoming yogis.

The IYI grew through word of mouth and it continued to grow. New institutes opened up all over the country and, eventually, all over the world. Gurudev received many invitations to give public talks. He spoke at churches, colleges, conferences, and festivals and on radio and television. He gave a number of talks at Horizon House, a treatment center for drug addicts, where IYI teachers taught Yoga full time. He was even invited to speak at prisons.

Lorton Complex, a federal prison in Virginia, near Washington, DC was one. The invitation came with a pretty remarkable story.

One of the prisoners had become a student of Integral Yoga and a devotee of Gurudev about a year before being incarcerated at Lorton Complex. It was in the late 60s that this young man had been arrested in Washington, DC for selling ten pounds of hashish. Able to post bail immediately, he avoided incarceration while his case was being handled in court. The court case moved along slowly and, in the meantime, he became interested in a woman who started taking him to Gurudev's talks at the Universalist Church in Manhattan. Really, he went along because of his interest in the woman, but he was inspired by what Gurudev was saying and he especially admired Gurudev's equanimity.

He continued going to the talks and began practicing *Hatha Yoga*. In court, though, he kept losing appeals and, finally, he lost the case. On the other hand, as his court situation worsened, his Yoga practice improved. Although part of him still resisted and didn't want any help, his awareness was expanding. The turning point for him came when, at the end of the summer, he took *mantra* initiation (a ceremony held when one becomes a disciple of a guru and is given a particular *mantra*, or sacred sound, to use for meditation) at an Integral Yoga retreat. The experience was profound and transformative, with old negative thoughts and habits falling away. The following year, when he'd completely lost the connection with his old way of life, he was ready to pay his karmic dues. The judge sentenced him to two to six years in prison, and he had to pay a $10,000 fine.

This yogi was sent to Lorton Complex and was placed, at first, in the maximum security facility. He managed to keep his *mala* (rosary) and was able to do *Hatha Yoga* next to his bed. For three weeks, he had no contact with the outside world and would have gone mad had he not decided to concentrate on writing a poem in Sanskrit for Gurudev. He used a Sanskrit dictionary to translate, word for word, the poem that he'd written in English. He had to focus really hard in order to copy the unfamiliar Sanskrit characters correctly. What kept him sane were the hours of intense concentration. Meanwhile, his cellmate, a bank robber, watched him practicing meditation and *Hatha* postures. Soon, he began to ask questions; and then, he too, began doing the postures.

Before long, the yogi was given an office job and moved to a dormitory with a hundred other men. Not only did he continue his own Yoga practices, but he began teaching others, and a group of ten inmates began meeting twice a week in the prison chapel, once a week for *Hatha Yoga* and once a week for *satsang* (spiritual gathering) and discussion.

The yogi was also in touch with a member of the Washington Integral Yoga Institute and managed to arrange for this man to teach Yoga, once a week, in the prison. Then, Gurudev came to visit. Everyone, almost a hundred men, helped to organize the event. Gurudev told them:

"Thank you for inviting me. I am happy to be here. Yes, I am aware that I am in a place where people come to be corrected. It is something like a repair shop, where things are restored to their proper shape. That means that you are supposed to be in a particular shape and, somehow, you have gotten out of that shape. You were once well-formed, somehow you got de-formed, and now you have to be re-formed.

"So, don't think that anyone is punishing you. The intention is not punishment; the intention is to help you to return to your original state. And don't think that this is the only reformatory. The entire world, itself, is a correctional institution. All through life, we slip from our original state and are reformed, again and again.

"How did we slip from our original state? By our own thinking. Through wrong thoughts, our minds become disturbed. We lose our peace. Question your mind: Why am I disturbed? You may try to put the blame on someone else. But that is not the right answer. If we really analyze, ultimately, we will come to this one truth: we just wanted something for ourselves. Most crimes are committed for the sake of this selfishness. If only we could get rid of that selfishness and think in terms of the whole world, then the mind would become pure and peaceful.

"Make use of this opportunity. Don't send out undesirable thoughts of hatred or resentment. There is no need for it. Suffering is to be accepted. Accept it and purge out all the sins accumulated by your past deeds, whether yesterday's or yesteryear's or yesterlife's.

"Many have done this. I have visited many correctional institutions and I see this everywhere. If even one person in an institution gets interested in Yoga, through that one, more and more will get interested and get benefited. So set an example. Then, you can walk out as well reformed, beautiful people–peaceful and useful to the entire community."

After the talk, Gurudev blessed his devotee, encouraging him to continue the fine work. Eventually, this man was moved to a minimum security facility where he was granted permission to leave every Friday evening to attend *Raja Yoga* classes at the Washington DC IYI. Nevertheless, during this time, life became challenging, as his diet was poor and there were several setbacks in his court motions for release from prison. However, at the height of this disciple's depression, Gurudev came, again, to speak this time at the minimum security prison. According to him, Gurudev's "radiance and love energized everyone." He, himself, was able to pull out of the depression and use his energy and talents positively to serve others. He became a successful international business man, married and helped to raise a beautiful family.

Upheaval and Transformation

When Gurudev arrived in the United States in 1966, the socio-political atmosphere in the US was explosive, literally and figuratively. President John F. Kennedy had been assassinated in November of 1963. In February of 1965, the US began bombing North Viet Nam and using jet fighters inside South Viet Nam. In the same month, Martin Luther King, Jr. and 770 other civil rights activists were arrested in Selma, Alabama and Malcolm X was shot and killed in a Harlem auditorium. Large quantities of the hallucinogenic drug LSD became available, and draft-card burning became a federal offense. Several Buddhist monks in Viet

Nam immolated themselves to protest the ongoing and relentless war. There were uprisings in African-American neighborhoods, innumerable anti-war demonstrations, and the emergence of the Black Power movement. In early March, the first American soldier "officially" stepped onto the battlefield in Viet Nam. As Bob Dylan observed, the times they were a-changin'. There were, in fact, two concurrent revolutions: the flower-power revolution of the rebellious white middle-class young people, who sought freedom from convention and tradition, and the black-power revolution of frustrated young African Americans, who sought freedom from hundreds of years of racial oppression.

It was a time of exhilaration and change—the first landing on the moon, the Beatles, and Charles Evers of Fayette, Mississippi, elected the first black mayor of an integrated southern community—but it was also a time of hostility and profound tragedy: the assassinations of Martin Luther King, Jr. and Robert F. Kennedy and the violent police actions on college campuses, resulting in the wounding and killing of many non-violent anti-war student demonstrators. There was violence on the streets, on college campuses, in courtrooms, and in prisons. It was during this turbulent period that Gurudev was invited to speak at Soledad Prison in California. The October 1, 1973, issue of the prison newspaper, the *Soledad Star News*, reported the event:

"Remember the flick *Woodstock*? OK. Remember the man with the flowing robes and the long white beard? His name is Swami Satchidananda and he was the guest of the Yoga Group in the Protestant Chapel this past Thursday evening. Or maybe it was that we were his guests. In any event, the meeting was one memorable occasion for the men who were fortunate enough to attend.

"Active members of the regularly scheduled *Hatha Yoga* group will well remember the tape-recordings played of the Swamiji's talks, which were given at some of his other appearances, but to hear this man of true peace speak before you, to sit in his presence, well, because of just such an opportunity, many inmates have now had the chance to know a genuine sense of serenity, as exemplified by the Swamiji. In every interpretation of the word, this writer has finally come to know what is meant by expressing love for one's spiritual master!

"The evening activity began not upon his arrival, but weeks in advance, when it was first learned that the North Facility Yoga Group would be blessed with his presence. The feelings felt last Thursday were not unlike those of two, long separated family members who've at last found one another. Instant recognition and relief.

"As Swamiji and his entourage passed through the Control Patio-Area, en route to the Chapel, all eyes fixed upon the long, flowing orange and yellow robes (symbolizing celibacy and service to others), while he casually, and with an air of humble, almost invisible gait, crossed the Patio-Area as you or I would cross the Yard—as if he were meant to be here and were one of us."

Indeed, what the *Soledad Star News* reporter was sensing was that Gurudev felt like one of them, because—as Gurudev perceived it—we are in fact, all one. Established in peace and unconditional love, he had no fear and felt at home everywhere. That evening in September, Gurudev gave the following talk to the members of the Soledad Prison's North Facility Yoga Group.

Soledad Prison
Soledad, California, September 20, 1973

Ups & Downs

I wonder how I should begin. Should I say that I am happy to see you all or that I am sorry to see you all? I kind of have mixed feelings.

Certainly, I am not happy to see you all here. At the same time, I am happy to see that you are all interested in Yoga, in making your life more beautiful. So, I am here sitting with mixed feelings. In fact, the very life, itself, is mixed. You are not always happy and you are not always unhappy. Life means ups and down. Even when you walk toward something, you have to use both the right and left legs; one goes forward and one stays behind. Constant contrasting movements

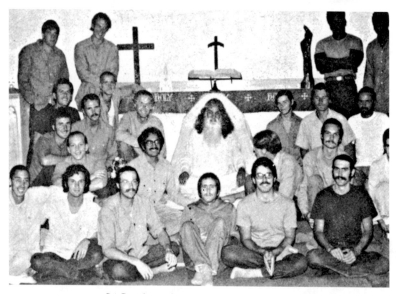

Sri Gurudev with members of Soledad Prison's North Facility Yoga Group.

make us go far. That, itself, is a small clue for us to know how to proceed, between the ups and downs, toward our goal.

Without the ups and downs, life is meaningless. Even in school, sometimes they teach us, other times they examine us. When we are learning, our teachers give us all their cooperation; and when we make mistakes, they correct us. But when we are in the examination hall, they refuse to help us. In the classroom, when you ask a question, the teacher will immediately answer. But in the examination hall, they won't. Why? Because they are really testing your capabilities; they are testing how much you have learned from the classroom. Life also is like that. Sometimes we learn and sometimes we are tested on our learning. If we understand life well, we won't be upset over all these changes. At any given moment, we will understand that moment very well, we will make use of it and we will grow further. That is the aim of Yoga, also.

Probably, you might have heard about Yoga, apart from the yogic physical postures. Yoga is not just a few physical postures, and it is not, as some of your administrative officers call it, acrobatics–they warned us ahead not to have any acrobatics here. I can't blame them for calling it acrobatics, because that is mostly the way Yoga is presented, as just something physical. For instance, some people say that if you stand on your head for an hour you are a great yogi. But I have a different way of thinking about it. I tell people that even before you try to stand on your head, you should learn to stand on your feet well. Without even knowing how to stand on our own feet, what's the use of standing on our head?

Life is a Correctional Institution

Take life easy, understand it well; make use of it well. In a way, don't think that this is the only place that is called a prison or a correctional institution. Sometimes, it even makes me laugh when I am told that this is a correctional institution. Tell me a place where you are not corrected. From the very birth to the very death, you are constantly corrected, is it not? Your papas and mamas corrected you. In the classrooms, your teachers and professors correct you. Even the highways correct you. They ask you to stick to one lane and you are asked to follow certain routines, certain procedures. Every signboard corrects you. If you go to California, and if you are going in the wrong direction, the signboard says: "This way goes to Utah, not to California. Turn around." This means that you become disciplined.

Actually, the entire life is a learning experience and the whole world is a correctional institution until we get corrected. As long as we make mistakes, we need correction. So correction is not something that you call punishment. Even doctors correct you. A psychologist corrects you when some of the screws in your head become loose. They correct you, tighten up all the screws. When something goes wrong with some of the organs, physicians correct you; they cure you. Likewise, the experience in this institution is also a form of curative procedure.

So, why do we need correction? Because we make mistakes. The one who doesn't make any mistakes doesn't need any correction. Somehow, though, we all learn by our mistakes. Nobody has ever learned anything without making mistakes. That's why there is a maxim, saying, "Failures are nothing but stepping stones for your future success."

Every mistake is a stepping stone. You learn by your mistakes, and then you go further. In that sense, we are all in some kind of prison or other. In fact, even living in the very body, itself, is a prison. The body itself is a prison to us because, as souls, we are limited within this body. We are restricted. We can't reach beyond our own limit. But as spirit, as the soul, we can reach much further. However, the spirit, the soul, is limited within the body. So, how can we regulate our life, how can we discipline it, how can we use it well? Actually, life, itself, is disciplined. There is a discipline everywhere. Look at anything in this world, animate or inanimate, and you'll see discipline at work. The entire universe is disciplined. Look at the sun; look at the moon; look at the stars. They don't just move as they want. They are all controlled by a cosmic law, controlled by absolute discipline. Otherwise, we would not be able to figure out exactly when the sun will dawn on a given date. What's more, all our space projects would be utter failures if they just ran anytime they wanted. Do you see? A spacecraft takes off at a certain given minute, because the experts figure out, after so many days of analysis and calculation, that at exactly such and such hour, such and such minute, the spacecraft will land on such and such a spot on the moon. How is it possible? Because all the planets move according to a particular law. What would happen, for example, when the spacecraft left the earth and before it reached the moon, if the moon, all of sudden, thought, "I have been following the same discipline every day and I'm a little bored; why don't I just take a little rest?" and it stopped spinning for a couple of hours and then started moving? Your lunar landing module would land somewhere different from the place where it was expected to land. That means that there is discipline everywhere.

This example illustrates that whoever follows the discipline set by nature's law will experience a smooth journey in his or her life. But when we make mistakes, when we disobey the law of nature, then we come across difficulties, troubles. And the very nature, itself, corrects us by way of suffering. Take, for example, eating, a simple process that we do daily. If we don't eat the right food, at the right time, and by the right method, then our stomach gets into trouble. However, if we follow nature's law, eating the right food, in the right way, and in the right quantity and quality, then the stomach digests and assimilates the food well and we get enough nourishment.

On the other hand, if we make a mistake, we get the ache, the stomachache. And then the doctor has to correct it. So the ache of the stomach is a kind of suffering to the stomach. This is just one example. It is like this whenever we make any kind of mistake. That is, we face the result of the mistake as a kind of suffering, a punishment, if you want to call it that way. But that punishment doesn't come out of any hatred. The stomach aches not because the stomach hates us. The stomach is only telling us that we made a mistake and that we have to correct that mistake. It is saying, "Wait! Don't eat any more until I correct the mistake."

So, the aches and pains are good signs; they are warnings for us to know that there is something wrong somewhere and that we should get the problem corrected. To correct the problem, you could call a doctor. And would you say that the doctor is punishing you when he gives you a purgative? No. But if we don't understand this process, then everything becomes a big burden, everything is unwanted; however, if you understand it, then you can make the best use of the situation.

By the way, when I go to a correctional institution like this I tell the people that I had a friend who said that you appreciate being called "convicts." Is that correct? Not "inmates"? Am I right? Well, it is only a different name, but, somehow, "inmates" feels like a better term. But it all depends upon how you feel. In any case, I always tell inmates that a correctional facility is not a place of punishment, a place of ordeal, since you are not here because the authorities or the judges or the lawyer or whoever it may be hated you. Probably, they saw that you did something wrong, that you disobeyed a certain law of nature (it need not always be man's law). After all, what is man's law? Man's law should agree with nature's law. Man makes laws according to nature's law. When we violate that law, we hate ourselves and others also and we are treated for that. So this institution is a treatment center. Furthermore, I always tell inmates that they don't even need to wait for the authorities to treat them;

they can treat themselves. In a hospital, for example, what the doctor does is very little. But the patient can do a lot to cure him- or herself. That is where the proper understanding comes in. In fact, I always say that a correctional institution is a kind of monastery. It is a place for penance. And I should say that, in a way, you are fortunate in having a place of penance like this. Why? You are well protected from unnecessary disturbances. You are given doctors and certified food, and even a Swami cannot come disturb you; he has to pass through so many gates. You are well protected. And what is it that they are protecting? They are protecting your seclusion.

The Law of *Karma*

You are here doing penance, meditation. You've been given the opportunity to make use of this time to correct yourself, to reform yourself. Some of you might think, "Well, I haven't done anything. By certain false witnesses, certain prejudices, I have been brought here, but I have not done anything." This may be true. It's not that every one of you here has really committed some crime and that's why you are here. Maybe due to some false witnesses or some prejudice, you might have been convicted without even a proper reason. There are cases like that. Even to them I say, there cannot be a reaction without an action. The very fact that you are here means that there is a reaction to some of your past actions. Or, in plain language, you might not have done anything to put yourself into this prison now, but you might have done something before and escaped from that. The law of *karma*, or nature's law, is that you can't escape from your actions. You may escape from man's judgment but never from God's judgment.

To make an analogy, say that the two of us go to a restaurant where we overeat, maybe because some dish was especially delicious. One of us gets a stomachache immediately. The other person doesn't get anything but, after three days, she also gets sick. She should not say, "But I did not eat anything special yesterday. Why should I get a stomachache?" She forgot that three days before, she overate.

This analogy means that certain results take time to come to the surface. That is the law of *karma*: every action has its reaction.

It is only a question of time. So, ten years before, you might have committed a crime and, somehow, you escaped from man's law. After ten years, without even having committed any crime, you are brought in. In that case, you have to understand: "Yes; I escaped then, but God took time to punish me." Again, punishment doesn't mean that God hated us or that the authorities or the judges hated us. No. They are trying to purge out our wrong actions, like the doctor trying to give a purgative, so that the poisons that we consume will come out. Therefore, this situation is a purgative. And what is it a purgative for? It is a purgative that will make our system become cleaner and purer, so that we can eliminate all the toxins. Physically, the toxins are eliminated to keep the body healthy. Mentally, the sins are eliminated to keep the mind healthy. When we're referring to the physical, we talk about "toxins"; when we're referring to the mental, we talk about "sins." And what do we mean by "sin"? Sin is a violation of nature's law. If we accept it that way, we will make the best use of this place. Because, after all, what do all the scriptures, all the religious teachings tell us? They tell us to be pure, to keep ourselves clean and pure. And they tell us that the goal is peace.

Naturally, we are all interested in peace and happiness. But we can never be happy with an unclean mind or with a sickly body. So, the goal is to keep the body clean and the mind calm. That is what Yoga teaches. That is why when you practice some of the Yoga postures, the goal is to free your body from the toxins so that you can eliminate the tension. The body becomes lighter, more relaxed and it gets rejuvenated. In the same way, by following certain moral precepts, by developing faith in God, devotion, our mind becomes more and more quiet and calm. We free our mind from all the undesirable actions, the undesirable thinking.

Blessed are the Pure

By the way, are you all Christians or Catholics, and are there any Jewish people here? What is the faith that you believe in? Do you have faith? What is your faith? Protestant? Catholic? Oh, mostly Christian, I see. So you believe in the Bible then? What does the

Bible say? It says that even to see God, one should be pure. "Blessed are the pure in heart. They shall see God." Without the purity, God cannot be seen. And where is that God? God is within you. God is everywhere, so God is within you too. Therefore, it should be easier to see God within than outside. But to see the God within, you must have a peaceful, pure mind. With an impure mind you cannot see God. God is in you as peace, as joy. Take this rose, for instance. Could I see the real color of this rose if my eyes were jaundiced? No. Why? Because when my eyes are jaundiced, I will see a yellow rose, not a pink rose. I will say, "What a pretty yellow rose," and you will laugh at me. To me, what I see is right. Why? Because I see a yellow rose. Unfortunately, I forgot that my eyes are not clean. With a jaundiced eye, you see everything as yellow. With a clear eye, you can see the right color. So, if I could change the wording in this connection, I would say, "Blessed are those that have a clear eye; they shall see the rose in its color." In the same sense, we could say, "Blessed are the people who have a clean mind, a pure mind; it is only those people who can see God's real form, as peace and joy."

In fact, this advice, or this requirement is what you find in every scripture, not only in the Bible. The Buddhist scriptures say so. The Hindu scriptures say so. Yoga puts it in plain language: keep your mind calm and you see everything as beautiful. You see everything. You see the truth.

Now, again, how does one get that purity of mind? The question might be: Can I make my mind pure? To that I say: You don't need to make your mind pure. By nature your mind is pure. You are born with a pure mind. Look at a baby. How peaceful it is; how happy it is. Can you see any impurity in the mind of a baby? What a charming face. When you were born, every one of the neighbors came to hug you, to give you a kiss. "What an angel, a darling." But what happened to that angelic face, that darling face now? See, you are born beautiful; you are born with an angel face, a clean calm mind. But somehow, slowly, it all got distorted. It's like buying a new item of clothing from the store. When you buy the item, the cloth is new, fresh and clean. But, when you start wearing it, slowly, dust and dirt start accumulating. And if you don't wash the clothing, the dirt starts building up, coat upon coat. The same thing happens to our mind. We allow all the dirty things to come into the mind, making it unclean. So, what should we do to remove the dirt from clothing or, analogously, from the mind, so that they become shiny and clean, again? You do what you would do with a mirror that is coated with dust. You clean it. When the mirror is coated with dust, you see only a distorted reflection. After the mirror has been cleaned, you see the beautiful reflection, again. We all still have that beautiful mind. Somehow we just allowed it, by our own negligence, our own carelessness, to get distorted.

And that is why, a little while ago, I used the word "reformation." But what do we mean by reformation? "Re-formation," is it not so? And why do you want to reform? You want to *reform* because you were in the proper *form* before, when you were a baby. Then, you got *deformed*. Now, you have to be *reformed*. Logically, if you haven't allowed yourself to be deformed, then there's no need for you to reform. So we just slipped from our position and we have to go back to that. And that is where all the religious practices and all the Yoga practices help us. They help us in reforming the body and mind. That means that they help us to remove all the dirt, both the physical and mental dirt.

To put it briefly, physical dirt is caused by improper eating, by putting improper things into the body, and I'm not talking only about solid food. Liquids also go into the body, and if we don't drink the right liquids, the body gets affected. Furthermore, if we don't inhale the right air, the body also gets affected. What a beautiful countryside this is. You get fresh air, is it not so? A lot of fresh air. There is no pollution in this area. You are really lucky. While living in this environment of unpolluted, fresh air, which is free for you, you can inhale as much as you want. They're not going to charge you. However, do you always do that? No? Only those who practice Yoga take a deep breath, right? But even the others, even those who don't take deep breaths, still inhale a little of the free, fresh air. Unfortunately, some of those people inhale a lot of some other kind of air, also. Which air is that? The air that is filled with nicotine.

Again, to purify your lungs, fresh, free air is given to you, without even any charge. Yet, you don't want to inhale that good air any more. You want to inhale nicotine. Why do you do it? Is it not a sin? When God has given you fresh, free air, a free gift, you don't want it. Instead, you want to char your lungs with nicotine. That means that you are violating nature's law. Certainly, for that sake, you have to face the reaction. Is that not correct? So, nature punishes you with a little cough or sneezing and then, later on, a little lung trouble. And the Surgeon General should warn you. But, actually, the Super Surgeon has already warned you.

Smoking is just one example of how we pollute our system by our own wrong habits. That is why Yoga tells you, "Take care of your body: eat the right food, drink the right liquids and inhale the right air. Then, you won't be putting any more toxins into the system." And if there are any toxins already in the system, eliminate them by doing some Yoga.

Certainly, by now, you are enjoying the benefit of Yoga, how relaxing it is. You must be feeling really very light–no tension anywhere physically. And, as for cleaning the mind, there's some good advice, too: Stay away from wrong thinking. Think good things. Read nice books. See the right things. Stay away from dirty thoughts. Keep the mind free. Lead a little more selfless life. Be dedicated. Be useful to people. At the same time, be a little more thankful to people also for all the gifts they have given us and for all the kind acts they have done. This is all Yoga and this is the same guidance that all religions offer. When we learn to live that way, then we feel that way. That is, we feel clear, our life becomes so easy and we have reformed ourselves. And, again, this correctional facility gives you the best opportunity to take this advice and practice this way of life.

Actually, you must, in a way, be thankful to the authorities and to all our friends, like Michael and the other friends, who have really come forward to help you by inviting these Yogis. In fact, Yoga is helping a lot. This is not the first correctional institution that I've visited. I visit many, many facilities; and, everywhere, the inmates seem to be getting really good benefits. I was introduced to this institution last September. One of you wrote to me, even before coming here, telling me, "This is where I am going," and he has been constantly writing, asking me to come. I am sure that you should be grateful to this one individual. It is mainly because of him that I came to know this place, Soledad. Then, we started sending people here. That's what. If there is one good man, many others get the benefit; and, then, through those others, more people benefit.

So, make use of this opportunity. Don't even send out any undesirable thoughts, thoughts of hatred or anything like that. I know that in many institutions, there is a kind of tension between the authorities and the inmates. There is no need for it. Suffering is to be accepted. Accept it. Think, "Well, God is giving me this suffering to purge out all my sins. Nobody can give me any kind of hardship; nobody can bring suffering to me. We are all only instruments." If you think in this way, then there is a nice understanding and good will. Think that they are all there to help you, that nobody is your enemy. This is just a way of thinking. Therefore, understand it properly, accept it and then purge out all your karmic sins. And when I say karmic sins, I mean all the sins that you accumulated by your past deeds, whenever those deeds were done. Be beautiful people. Be peaceful. Be useful to the community. And that is all I would like to tell you now.

At this point, maybe I can give some time to answering any questions that you might have. Do you want to ask anything? Ask me any questions, whatever you feel. Certainly, you would have gotten the answers within. And, probably, by the time I come again next time, I won't be seeing many of you. I don't want to see you. But if, by any chance, a few still remain, by your example I want you to inspire many of the people who live here, the convicts. Somehow, my speech doesn't want to come out to say "convicts." Somehow, I feel that "convicts" is not the right term. The "members of the institute," I'll put it that way.

In any case, I'm happy to see that so many of you came to this talk today. The same thing happened when I went to Lorton Prison near Washington, DC. The first time, a small group came. When

I went the second time, the hall was full. Why? Because they got inspired by those who came the first time. So, that is another thing that you can do. You can talk to all your fellow members, telling them how nice, how beautiful the experience was. Let this be a good opportunity for them to know a little. In fact, some of the members who got out of Lorton Prison are now in charge of my centers. In Washington, DC, for example, the Integral Yoga Institute is headed by a boy named Jay. We call him Jay. He does beautiful silk screen work. He even made tee shirts there. Jay was at Lorton Prison. Imagine. That is what I would want to see. When you come out, probably each one should go out and start a Yoga center. Set an example. Let people know that you really got the benefit here. You shouldn't go with any kind of hard feeling.

Let's answer some questions now.

Re-formation

Question: I sometimes have difficulty justifying my experience in this institution, that is, in terms of "corrections," as you used the word. I can understand what you mean when you say corrections. But I have a hard time saying to myself that this is really a correctional experience I'm into.

Sri Gurudev: Well, it's only terminology. Certainly, we all need corrections. Every minute, we are corrected. Are we completely free from any mistakes? We all make mistakes. We erred somewhere, sometime. And correction means reforming, taking away the mistake, like the doctor treating a patient because there is a disease, a disease that is either physical or mental. After all, what is disease? "Disease is that which caused you to lose your ease. Is it not so? You were at *ease*; all of a sudden, something happened, you did something and you lost your ease. Thus, you are *diseased*. Then, the doctor takes away the *dis*, putting you back at *ease*. So anything that marred our ease is to be taken out.

To repeat the analogy of the jaundiced eye, because I have too much bile in my liver, I see everything yellowish; the bile caused the yellowish color. When the bile is treated, I've cured myself of the jaundice and I see things clearly. So it's correctional. To rectify something is what you call correction. That is why I said that, sometimes, you may even feel that you have not done anything, that you are here by mistake. I have seen many cases like that. It's not that everybody who is here actually committed a crime. A couple of people, if they conspire well, can put you into any prison. Correct? Even an innocent person can be handcuffed easily. Nonetheless, to that person I say, "Don't blame them. They brought the conspiracy against you because you were fit for that. You did something before and escaped. Now the time has come and nature's law, God's law, brought a couple of people to incarcerate you. These individuals were only excuses. That is why without an action, there can never be reaction.

What you do, you pay for. Whatever you sow, you reap. If I sow something, you cannot reap it. You are the master of your destiny. So don't blame anybody at all. By unnecessarily blaming others, we create more hatred, more enemies. If you blame somebody else for your coming here and if you are really innocent, you will continue to blame that person, you will hate that person and what will you do the minute you walk out? You will look for that person, and you will raise your arm against him or her. "Dirty fellow, see I got out. Now, look; I am going to take revenge." You are going to do the same thing, again. Instead, I say: love that person. He or she has become only an excuse for you to come here. Your *karma* brought you here. Don't hate that person.

This is not just mere philosophy; it is a fact. If you had not done anything that would have brought you here, even if the whole world plotted against you, you wouldn't be here. I am positive about that. Our *karma*, our action, brings us a reaction. As I mentioned before, if I eat something nasty, something unfit, I must get a stomachache. If not, the law of *karma*, the law of action and reaction, cause and effect, will have no meaning. Human law may fail, but not God's law.

Action and Reaction

Question: Is not karma a form of revenge?
Sri Gurudev: The word "revenge" doesn't really bring a good meaning. Revenge means that you act out of hatred, that you want

to do something in return. *Karma*, on the other hand, is a form of purgation. It takes away the sins or the toxins that you put into the system. In Sanskrit, *karma* means action. Another meaning, though, is reaction. Thus, we say that by doing a *karma*, you face a *karma*; that is, action and reaction have the same name in Sanskrit.

So, an action brings a reaction. Therefore, you can't say that reaction means revenge for the action. Rather, the reaction is the product of the action, a process of cause and effect. "Revenge" means something different. When you take revenge on someone, the act is filled with hatred, with animosity. Doctors don't take revenge on you when they operate on patients. They put sharp knives into patients and cut. Sometimes, they even cut away limbs. Are doctors our enemies, then? No. They want to help us, and if nothing else can save us, doctors won't hesitate to cut away an arm or a part of the body if that can save us. In the same way, all reformation has that same purpose. Even our own pains have that purpose. Take, for example, a little fever. After all, what is fever? Fever is not a disease. It is your own built-in energy trying to burn out the toxins that you have put into the body by your wrong habits. So, fever is the effect of your body burning out the toxin; in other words, this process expresses itself as a fever. So, fever is a good sign. It helps you. So you can't say fever is taking revenge on you.

It's all in the Mind

Question: What is the karma of the officials who would try to reform inmates?

Sri Gurudev: Well, they must have done something, something good. That is why they have been chosen to help you. In a way, they too must have done something a little bad, had a little bad *karma*; otherwise, why should they come here and be within the compound to help you? They also have to be kept in with the lock and key. They also can't move around easily. In a way, they are also prisoners. They are within the compound, is it not? They don't have free movement either.

So, what is my *karma* now? Michael said, "I have to lock you in, Swami." That's my *karma*. Yes; they have been chosen for that purpose. They must have done something good. And cosmic law says: "You seem to be a good man. You can help them." That's why they are here, that is, if they have come with the idea of helping you. However, they might have come only to earn their livelihood, to make a few bucks, to buy their food, their bread, etc.

See, it's all in the mind. It's all a matter of how you accept it, how you think of it. In fact, with proper understanding, you can accept anything and everything, easily. Yes, proper understanding is necessary. In any situation, if you don't understand it, then it's a very tense one that's going to affect you. You won't like it. You will hate it. But the minute you try to understand it in the proper way, you will love it. Yes. For instance, take Michael who is here with us. He was in Lorton Prison. When he went into the prison, he hated it. He was so negative. He used to write letters to me, pouring out this negativity. But I wrote him back: "No; you are wrong. Be a yogi; understand the situation well." It took a little while for him to understand it. But, within a month, he changed his entire attitude. He became a wonderful person there. Everybody started liking him. He got more and more freedom and was able to go wherever he wanted. And then, very soon, he was able to go out. They gave him some time to go to get educated. He won the good will of people there. As a matter of fact, it is he who started the Yoga center there in the prison. That's what it all depends upon: how you see.

It's the same even in the family. If you see with a little suspicion, your own wife will be a deadly enemy to you. However, if you think of the day of your wedding—how beautiful she was and how lovely she looked at you and with what nice, loving eyes (or what lustful eyes) you saw her—if you think of that, your wife won't be an enemy to you then. That is to say, your enemy and your friend are within you. You make the hell and you make the heaven. It all depends on the way you look at it, on whether you have the proper relationship with anything and everything.

To give an example, you plug in a lamp and you get light, is it not? You plug in a tape recorder and you tape everything. You have the right relationship with electricity. However, if you plug in your fingers, you have the wrong relationship with it. You get a shock. Then you stand up and say, "How terrible it is! I don't want electricity here anymore. It's a terrible thing to have in the house." So, what about the others who plug in their lamps and get light? They will say, "What a fool you are. Electricity gives me light; it gives me music; it cooks my food. How dare you say it's dangerous, terrible?" Therefore, how can you say that electricity is good or bad? It's neither good, nor bad. It's just neutral.

If your approach is proper, it's good for you. If your approach is wrong, it's bad for you. In the same way, your son, your daughter, your wife, your mama, your papa, your officer and everybody, if you have the proper relationship with them, they are all wonderful to you. Your car, if you drive carefully, it is wonderful; it takes you to the goal. But if you allow somebody else to drive while you sit in the driver's seat—you know what I mean. Some people sit in the car, but they don't drive the car. Something within them drives the car and they become a menace on the road. In this case, we can't blame the car. That's what. It all depends upon how we accept things. To make the whole world a beautiful heaven, everybody will be our beloved friends, if you know how to deal with them properly. If we do not know how to deal with people properly, even your beloved mama would be a devil to you; in fact, nobody would be your friend then.

It's all a matter of our own projection. That is why I say that even before you pass judgment about the outside world—and about people—saying it's good or it's bad, judge yourself. "Am I good or bad? Am I judging properly? Do I have the authority to judge? Am I seeing things with clear eyes or am I prejudiced?" Suppose, sometime back, you got duped by a Swami like me, one with a long beard. The minute you see me, you'll think, "Here is another crook coming." Why? Because I might remind you of that man. You are biased. Your eyes are already coated with that prejudice, so everybody with a beard will look like the Swami you were deceived by. So, see without any prejudice. With clear vision, you see everybody as beautiful. You love everybody equally. That's why all we need is clear vision, a clean mind, and a clean body.

Even a handful of people like that, I think, would be enough. And you people, if you really, sincerely, take these things to heart and work along these lines, probably within a month, you will see that you will be able to inspire hundreds of people here. Even the authorities will look to you as someone totally different. They will; there is no doubt. You can claim that reverence from them just by your behavior.

No person is bad by birth. We are all really beautiful images of God, is it not? God made the human being in God's own image. Sometimes, though, by our own little weakness, we smear some dirt on ourselves, and we look a little ugly, that's all. Clean it off and we become beautiful again. You can earn the respect of everyone if you want it. Treat everybody equally. No difference whatsoever between one person and another. Whether the person is black or white or brown or yellow, rich or poor, we are all equal. We come from the same family. We are divine children. You are not in any way different from me. We are all one.

Sure, there may be a little difference between us in understanding, but all children go and tumble down into the mud and get smeared. Then, when they grow up, they keep themselves neat and clean. Maybe I gained a little experience myself by falling, by tumbling down, and now you are just learning. That is all the difference. Should I see you and look down upon you, saying, "I am great, but you are all this and that." That's why I always say to my Christian clergy friends, "Please don't call anyone a sinner; please don't say, 'You sinners!'" Nobody is a sinner in this world. Please let us forget that term.

We are all Divine Children

We make mistakes, but we are not sinners by birth. We are all divine children, born in the image of God. Accept that true entity. That is what Yoga is. And, again, Yoga is not anything different from your own faith. It is not a new religion. The same principles are taught in every religion. But, unfortunately, those fundamental truths seem to be ignored or forgotten by most of the followers. They just take the superficial differences and they fight between religion and religion. So, we have to go deep into the depths of our own religion and then we will see everybody as equal. Otherwise, what is the purpose or idea of looking up and saying, "Our Father in heaven." He is the Father of all of us. That means we are all equal, we are all one family. That should be our attitude. With that attitude, there will be beautiful harmony here between you all and the administration.

Sometimes, I feel so sorry seeing all kinds of troubles, revolts, hatred, and tension in institutions like this. There is no need for that. And I don't always blame the inmates. The authorities also should be blamed. I'm not only talking to you people, the inmates; I'm talking to them also. Whenever there is a row or trouble, is it just one-sided? Unless both hands come together, you can't make any noise. Is this not so? When you create the noise that comes from hitting the palms together, which palm will take the blame? Can the left palm say, "It is all the mistake of the right palm?" Then I would ask, "If he comes to try to hit you, why don't you go away? There won't be a noise then. Why should you stay right there? So, everyone should accept their mistake and correct it.

Vegetarianism

Question: Can you discuss vegetarianism?

Sri Gurudev: Well, do you have a choice here with respect to your meals? I'd like to know before I put forth a different kind of thinking. I don't want to bring in some kind of confusion. Probably, if a group of people want to be vegetarian, the institution should be able to provide you with that kind of food, right? It's not that every kind of food here contains meat. There are certain meatless foods, also. Take, for example, bread and butter. Do you get bread and butter? That's fine. Why say vegetarian food? We recommend vegetarian food, yes. In fact, all the scriptures recommend vegetarian food. No scripture has ever permitted you to eat meat. The Bible puts it clearly: God created nuts and fruits for you.

Apart from the religious point of view, even from the point of view of health, I would say that vegetables are less susceptible to disease, to germs, than are animals. And, also, there is the question of digestive power. You can digest your vegetables more easily than fat, than animal fat. But they may say that animal flesh has a lot of protein. However, the human body doesn't need that much concentrated protein. And you have protein in vegetables. Take, for example, soybeans. In fact, there are so many vegetarian foods that have protein. Most lentils, for instance, have plenty of protein, in a natural form and they don't leave many toxins in the system. On the other hand, animal fat contains cholesterol, because there is a lot of purine in animal fat. They may say, "You may not have enough strength if you eat only vegetables." Then, I would ask you to go to a zoo and ask the elephant about that. Elephants are vegetarians and they are the strongest animals. Where do they get all their strength? Just from leaves and grass.

It is a wrong notion that if you don't eat meat you become weak. Vegetarian food is the best food, even for the mind. Go to the zoo and look at all the carnivores. They are caged; they are restless, isn't that so? Their mouths smell awfully bad and their excretion smells bad. Then, go to see the cows, goats and horses. They'll smile at you. Their excretion doesn't smell bad. They are such peaceloving animals. Why? The diet makes the difference. The mind is more peaceful with vegetarian food. As for the body, carnivore bodies are foul-smelling. Why? Because of the meat that leaves a lot of toxins in the system. The system eliminates those toxins and when the toxins are eliminated, they come out with a lot of foul smell. For that reason mostly, the perspiration of people who eat meat smells awfully bad. So, some of those big companies who make all the antiperspiration things–what do you call them? Deodorants–make a lot of money. They tell you that however bad you smell, it doesn't matter; you can hide it. Take this and put it on to hide the smell. Yes, you can hide it, but you cannot clean it. The smell comes from within. They have advertisements where the man opens his mouth and talks to his beloved girlfriend. His breath is terrible until he uses a mouthwash to take away the bad smell. Why can't they tell you where that dirty matter comes from? Because they don't want to eliminate the cause. All they want to do is to hide the bad smell, to cover it up. In this case, you are putting everything under the rug. You are not cleaning the mouth.

Probably if enough people here say that they want some vegetarian food, certainly they should be able to make it. Until they do make it, though, just take some yogurt, bread, butter, nuts and cereals. Any kind of cereal is good. I think every menu will have something for you to eat. In fact, when I go to a restaurant, any restaurant, I just order whatever I want: some steamed vegetables, some bread and butter. I don't know what your normal menu is. What do you normally get?

Inmate: We usually have vegetables. We have fruit and cereal in the morning and meat at other meals.

Sri Gurudev: Cereal in the morning, vegetables and fruit, what else do you want? Just leave the other foods. I am particularly happy when I hear that beef prices are going up. Nowadays, in the market, you see a lot of imitation beef, made with soy, looking exactly like beef but made all in soy. It is very good. So, until you really make them have a vegetarian mess for you, you can just choose what you want. You don't need to eat all the different things. Sometimes on airplanes, even though I order vegetarian food, they forget and they bring me chicken with vegetables. I just take the chicken out and eat the rest. That is enough.

We Don't Need Brute Strength

We don't really need that much food. In fact, it's not how much you eat that is important. How you digest and assimilate the food is, actually, more important. We eat more than what we can digest. I work day and night. Twenty-five days of the month, I travel. Today, I am here, tomorrow somewhere in Dallas, the day after tomorrow somewhere on the East Coast. Then, the next day, I might be in London. I travel so much, I talk so much, I meet people and eat only once a day and that, too, just vegetarian food. I'm not tired. Not only do I visit and talk, but I also do manual work. I drive my car. Sometimes, you might see me driving a tractor at the *ashram*. I have enough strength. We don't need to be brutes. We don't need brute strength.

If you want to be strong and peaceful, eat fruit, nuts and vegetables instead of meat, and drink milk instead of rum. At the same time, instead of playing war drums, play some nice music, classical music. Then, you'll throw down your guns and you'll sit and meditate. It is the war drum and the rum that makes beasts of man. We don't need that animalistic tendency. We want to be human beings, more loving. I'm sure you can understand. Do you think that boys will fight without the war drum? No. War drumming makes them go crazy. Anybody, even a man who sits and meditates, when he hears the war drum, will get up and jump. It hypnotizes you. That is why we should choose our food, choose our reading materials and choose our music well. If we were peaceloving people, we would choose what makes us peaceful.

Peace won't come by itself if we don't take care of all our violence. The country talks so much about violence, violence, violence. At the same time, it educates even young children with plastic machine guns. "Rrrr," they go; and they say, "Papa and Mama, I kill you." That's how children learn. Then, when they grow up, they want real guns. Any minute that you turn on the TV, you hear a shot: Gunfire. And you see gunsmoke. And with all that, we don't want violence. Read any newspaper, turn on any radio, any TV, look at the toys; we can go and buy guns everywhere and then we talk so much about violence, violence, violence.

We don't do things properly. What is the need even for these prisons? There is no need. If we were not given the opportunities to commit crimes, we would all be good people. If I am given an opportunity, even I might be a rogue. So, put yourself in the proper environment and you will be powerful. That is the duty of the guards, also. Just as they protect you here, they have to protect the entire country. We need to have proper laws. For instance, there's so much permission, so much sanction given for drinking. The statistics say that more than 60 percent of automobile accidents are caused by drinking, by drunken drivers. And many of the murders, at least more than half, are caused by drunken people. At the same time, people say, "Have a nice drink. Come on, have a nice drink." On one side, it's, "Come on, drink." On the other side, because you were drunk, you committed a crime and got sent to prison. That is why there is a lot of weakness everywhere. And that is why: prevention is better than cure. But certainly, there is no need for me to tell you these things. Instead, I should be saying these things to those people who are sitting in the other prisons, like the prison that is called the Pentagon, etc., etc. This brings me to the subject of group *karma*.

Group *Karma*

As in the body, when parts of the body get contaminated, the entire body becomes septic. Then, trouble comes in. This is an analogy for what you call war. It's group *karma*. Take, for example, Hitler. Hitler put so many millions of Jewish people into the gas chambers. How do you explain that? It's their *karma*. Otherwise, why should God create a Hitler and permit him to do that? I ask this question to Jewish people. You believe in God and in His will. So, by whose will was Hitler born? And if everything is God's will, why should you hate Hitler? And why should you hate all the Christians? The Jewish people don't even want to repeat the name Jesus Christ. Why? Because of Christ, millions died. If you can have that much hatred, then you don't believe in God and in God's law. So that is why. But even though we accept God's law, that doesn't mean that we should take it for granted and just keep quiet. Somehow, something has happened, say, a clash started between two countries. In this case, the peace-loving people should come forward and do whatever they can. However, they should do it peacefully, because peace cannot be restored with violence.

Take, for example, the days when every university campus had a revolt. Why? They didn't want war in Vietnam. But could they stop the war in Vietnam by creating another war here? That's what. Violence can never be eliminated by violence. If that is what you're doing, you're contradicting yourself. If you don't believe in violence, you should not bring violence as an excuse in order to stop that violence. Many of these peace marches fail. Why? Because the people who are marching don't believe in peace. They talk of peace, but they are trying to achieve it through violence. All the peace talks fail because there is no peace in the minds of those involved. That's why people should not immediately resort to violence, wherever it is. Even in prisons, a lot of trouble is happening. Why? It's mistake on both the sides. We can never achieve anything by violence; that is certain. The world has never achieved anything through violence.

What about all these wars? What was the root cause of the Second World War? The root cause of the Second World War was that the First World War was not won properly. A victory in a war means, in the normal sense, that one country goes and throws bombs into another one, killing many people, and accepting the surrender of the rest of the people. Then, the so-called victors declare, "We won a victory." But that's not the real victory. They might have won, yes, but the remaining people will still have a grudge. Is it not so? And when those people rebuild their forces one day or another, they will start another war. To win a real victory is to win the hearts of those who were vanquished so that there won't be any loser. That is why World War I gave room for World War II and that is why World War II is giving room for World War III.

People always believe in violence, even in this arms race between Russia and America. Why? Both countries believe in arms strength. As long as you believe in arms strength, you can't achieve anything. You can control somebody out of fear for sometime, but even the weakest person will have an opportunity to throw a stone at you. Is it not so? So, the real winning is through love. That is how Jesus Christ, that is how Buddha won the whole world, not with a sword or gun, but with the heart. It is that victory that we want: love your neighbor; love your enemy. That is the best way to make him or to make her your friend.

Hatred will always beget hatred, whatever form it takes or wherever it may be. So, let us learn. It may not happen immediately. It will take time. But this is a positive way. By violence you may get something quickly, but it will be temporary, it won't last long.

Now let's do some *OM Shanti* chanting. *OM Shanti, OM Shanti, OM Shanti.*

Deuel Vocational Institute
Tracy, California, September 21, 1973

The first Integral Yoga Institute was founded on the Upper West Side of New York City in the spring of 1966. By the summer of 1969, several of Gurudev's devotees headed out to California,

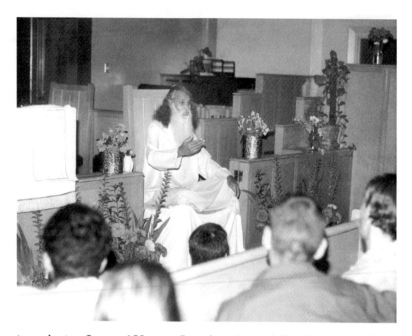

introducing Integral Yoga to Los Angeles and San Francisco. The organization continued to grow on both coasts. Ashrams opened in California, and in the fall of 1970, a second New York IYI opened its doors. Three years later, in April 1973, Satchidananda Ashram, Yogaville East officially opened its doors in Pomfret, Connecticut. By the 1970s, a number of Integral Yoga teachers on both coasts were bringing Integral Yoga and the teachings of Gurudev into prisons, and they were instrumental in bringing Gurudev into the prisons to meet their students in person. In fact, on September 21, 1973, a day after he spoke to the men at Soledad Prison, Gurudev visited Deuel Vocational Institute, a correctional institute in the San Francisco Bay area. This talk focused on the more philosophical aspects of Yoga.

Getting into that Original Nature

Beloved friends, I am really delighted to know and to see that the idea of Yoga is penetrating even behind electronically locked doors. If Yoga is really going to be useful, this should be the place for it. I don't call this a correctional institute; rather, I would like to call this a Yoga institute, because Yoga could be achieved only when you correct yourself. Yoga is always there. In reality we are all yogis. Well, this makes me realize that before I go any further, I should remind you then what Yoga is. If not, it doesn't make any sense to tell you that we are all yogis.

Yoga is not just something where you perform certain breathing techniques or stand on the head for a while. Even though that is part of Yoga, the real Yoga means to express your own divinity, your own true self. How? By keeping your mind well balanced. That's why the very definition of Yoga in the yogic scripture is "equanimity of mind," *samatvam yoga ucyate*. What the scripture says is that Yoga is equanimity of mind–totally tranquil, well balanced, not getting off balance. And this balance need not be brought in afresh. In fact, no balance can be brought in. Everything in nature is already balanced; if we leave it undisturbed, then it is balanced. Take a bowl of water. If we don't disturb it, it is balanced. It remains calm and quiet. For that is its natural state, that is the original state. You can call it the divine state. That's why we seek God, because God is well balanced. God is pure, calm, serene. God is above all these dualities.

So, getting into that original nature of being peaceful, being tranquil, well balanced is what you call the yogic state. That's why I said that by nature we are all balanced. Furthermore, the scriptures also remind us that we were all created in the image of the balanced one: God. God made the human being in God's own image. And what is the image of God? Well balanced, totally pure, perfect. A perfect Creator could never create an imperfect, off-balanced image. So, in a sense, we are that divine image. That is the truth but, fortunately or unfortunately, after having created us in God's image, God gave us a little freedom, freedom to think any way we want. You can think yourself well balanced, resting in your own true nature, or you can think yourself to be a little off balance. We have been given that freedom. As you all know, the proverb says, "As you think, so you become."

Earlier, our revered Chaplain gave me a few moments to be in his room, and I opened a book there and saw a quote from Shakespeare. It said: "There is nothing good or bad." The essence of this idea is that there is nothing that is good or bad; rather, it is all up to you; you become good or bad, as you think. If you think good, it is good; if you think bad, it is bad. That's what I always say, that it depends on the approach, on your relationship with things. As a matter of fact, there is nothing good or bad in this entire cosmos. Nothing. Nobody can pinpoint anything and say, "This is bad; we should not have this on the surface of the earth." But anything can become good or bad, according to your approach, according to your relationship with it.

Let me give you a simple example that will help you understand. I'm going to ask you a question. Electricity is something that we always have, for example, we have the electricity outlet on the walls. Is electricity good or bad? And food: Is food good or bad? Who says it's good? Good, everybody agrees with him? No? What do you say? It's bad? So, now we have to vote, and the majority wins. How many of you want to say that electricity, the electrical outlet is good? I see that many hands are raised. And how many of you say it is bad? Now, fewer hands are raised. As for me, I would have to raise both hands. Is it good? Is it bad? It's neither. For if you just leave electricity unused, it is neither good nor bad to you. If you plug in a lamp, you get light. "See, the whole room is lit; how good it is." Plug in your radio and you get a wonderful music. But plug in your finger. Those who plug in their fingers say, "It's dreadful. No one should have electricity in the house. Cut all the wires. Start an anti-electricity campaign." We are used to starting all kinds of campaigns. And if these anti-electricity campaigners are clever in presenting their picture, they, too, can have a lot of followers. But the fact is that electricity, itself, is neither good nor bad. It becomes good if you approach it and use it in the proper way. However, if your approach is wrong, it becomes bad.

So, what is good and bad is not the electricity or the thing itself, but your approach to it. And that's what you call *thinking*, your
th   If you think well, it is good. If you do not think properly,
                verything in the world is like that. Take the motor car. Is
                ad? If you drive it safely, it is very good; it takes you to
ion. If you don't drive it well and you allow something

else, certain substances maybe, to get into you to drive you and the car, then the experience might turn out bad. When you fill the gas tank, maybe you also fill the bottle of spirituality. Yes, many people are spiritual drivers. They have a bottle of spirit, and they pour some spirituality into them and then drive the car, is it not? To these people, the car is a dangerous thing. It not only hurts them, but it also hurts others. Another example is deadly poison. Put it in the hands of a capable doctor, and he or she will use it to save your life. Put it in the hands of an ordinary person, it could be a killer. So, the same poison becomes a lifesaver at one point, and at another point it destroys life. Thus, you cannot label poison as bad or good, because God created that poison, too.

With respect to the one who is fully balanced, who is neither good nor bad, who is above both (we say that person resides in the Absolute), that person doesn't swing to any side; there's no leaning to any side. He or she *is*, that's all. As such, we are all the products of that Absolute. But, as I said before, somehow, we have been given a little freedom to think any way we want. So, we imagine ourselves to be this or that. And the more you imagine, the more you become that. As you think, so you become. Therefore, in the name of Yoga, we ask people to have right thinking. Think the right way. Learn to keep a proper relationship with everything. First think about the positive side by staying away from the negative side, and then, from the positive side go to the neutral level. That is, you don't even get caught in the positive either. You are going toward the positive just to get rid of the negative. And then, from the positive, you come to the neutral level, to the zero point. Only then can you become a perfect instrument, a useful and a peaceful person. Only then are you fit to judge others, to serve others.

Take the case of a balance, a weighing machine. Imagine that you are a weight watcher. You go into the bathroom, stand on the scale and, all of a sudden, you feel horrible. "What is this: 168 pounds? I was only 140 last night." You jump out of balance; then, you look for the accuracy of the balance itself. Then, to your own satisfaction, you notice that the balance has lost its zero point and has moved about 28 pounds to one side. Somebody must have meddled with the knob there, a little screw loose somewhere. So, what do you do to know your correct weight? You set the balance to the zero point again, is it not? You correct it. There you are; you're doing the job of a correctional institute authority and that machine is being corrected. Once you set the needle to the zero point, when you step up again on the scale, you see your old weight of 140 pounds. Therefore, when does the balance, the scale, show you the correct weight? When the dial remains at the zero point. It's neither negative nor positive, neither plus nor minus. Isn't it so? That's Yoga, to find the neutral point, what we call the peaceful point, the tranquil point, the balanced state.

A balanced person will not lean to any side. He will not be prejudiced by anything, neither by good nor bad. She will keep her mind cool. Unfortunately, nowadays, people seem to want to give you that "cool" with a couple of extra long millimeters [of a cigarette]. "Kools; make yourself cool; it's naturally refreshing." You don't need any outside help to come back to your cool state. There's a double zero in "cool," right in the middle. That's why even God remains in that middle zero. The middle point of God is an "o," is it not? G-O-D. The middle, central point of God is zero, "O." "O" means zero, either nothing or full—complete—correct? The "o" is a complete circle; there are no ends; it's total. Or, it could be a complete zero. You neither go to nothing, nor do you go to everything. Both ends meet. That is the yogic state. You might say, "Well, by being in that state, what am I going to do?" "Am I going to be useful?" You don't need to worry about it. Even the very worry will make you off balance. You don't need to be worrying about that.

Take, for example, the plant. The flower didn't worry when it was on the plant: "What am I doing here, sitting on the plant. Why doesn't somebody cut me and put me on the altar? The Swami is coming." The flower didn't say anything. It didn't worry; it was just there, calm and cool and serene and composed. You looked at it, thinking, "That's a really nice flower. Let me put it on the altar." So, okay, you cut it, you put it on the altar, and is it excited now, jumping and dancing? No. It's still retaining its coolness. It's just there. Wherever it is, it is. It remains calm, but we are using it. It is not excited, but we are excited over these beautiful decorations. The flower serves us by just being. It doesn't demand, "Come on; make use of me. I am here; I've already bloomed; I'm waiting for you." No. Everything in nature is like that. It is just there, it *is*. God *is*, nature *is*, the fruit *is*, the flower *is*. In the same way, by just living that way, you become a really wonderful person. You become useful. Whoever knows your value will use you. You don't need to worry about it. They will come after you. When a tree is laden with fruit, it never sends an invitation to the bats, does it? All the bats run after the fruit. When the flower is laden with honey, without any invitation, the bees come there. Our purpose is to find that neutrality, that equanimity, that tranquility by correcting our screws and nuts if they're loose, to tighten them a little.

To make another analogy, which machines go to the garage, which go to the repair shop? All those that got worn out a little or that got loosened. We are all like that. If we recognize that, who will invite a doctor in? Only people who know that they are sick. They should first recognize that they need correction; then, they will ask someone to come and correct the condition. If we can understand this well, we won't have any negative feelings about institutions like this one. We all need correction, whether it is within an institution or outside of one. In fact, the entire world is a correctional institute. Don't think that this facility is the only place. No matter where we are, our own conscience is within us, watching us. You can lie to another person, you can spend your money in getting the service of able lawyers, you can get away from man's law; but your own conscience laughs behind you and says, "Can you get away from me? No. You wait; I'm going to do that. I'm only marking the right time." That is God in you, warning you, correcting you. So, whoever listens to that God within prevents him- or herself from falling into temptations, from getting into trouble.

Prevention is better than cure. But some do not listen to that advice, they just ignore it and they act. Then, they face the reaction, which comes as a kind of suffering that you may call punishment. But it's not that somebody else comes to punish you. Your own wrong action brings a reaction with certain suffering, which you may call punishment. For instance, your stomachache is the punishment for your wrong eating. Then why are you punished? Not because someone or something hates you. A doctor performs a very painful operation on you. Can you say that the doctor is punishing you? He is trying to squeeze out the toxins, the pus that has formed in your system and that causes suffering.

Thus, punishment is not something that comes because the other person hates you; instead, the other person loves you. That is the reason why, even in the Bible, Lord Jesus said, "If you want to follow me to the Kingdom of Heaven, carry the Cross." Carrying the cross means: accepting suffering. Even if you are crucified, accept it. Think that some of your karmic actions are being purged out, that some of your wrong reactions are being removed. You are being cleared so that you can come back to that neutral state of equanimity. That is what you call the Yoga state.

Now, at this point, I would like to go to another area. What is the reason for our wrong thinking, for our losing the balance? It's mainly because we have forgotten our own true nature. We have forgotten that the peace and joy are always within. Because the peace and joy are always within, we don't seem to turn inward to see, to realize what is within us. Instead, we allow our senses to go outward, to become extroverted. So, we miss what is within and we look for it from outside, thinking, "By getting that, I'll be happy; by getting this, I'll be happy." It's just like running after your own shadow. We run after happiness, thinking that it comes from the outside.

When you try to hold on to something for yourself alone, you get anxiety, you worry because of the fear of losing the object of your desire. If only you knew that the happiness is within you, that you are that happiness, then you would never worry about getting anything or losing anything, because your happiness doesn't depend on that. You have realized your true nature. The minute you forget that, you become dependent on things; then, you are never independent. You may call yourself independent, free: "I'm a free person in a free country." Nobody is free. Only those who have realized their true nature, their true self, are really free people.

It is this freedom that is the goal of every scripture. *Liberation.*
Salvation. What do these words mean? *Freedom.*

Only the people who have attained salvation or liberation are
the really free people. Others are in prison, is it not so? When you
are not free, you are imprisoned. So, that is the prison then. Is it
within the walls? Behind the electronic doors? No. It is within you.
Your ignorance of your true nature is, itself, a prison; it's bondage.

Now, the issue is: theoretically, it seems to be all right. Yes, the
scriptures say, and the Swami also says, that we are all the image
of God, and we are happy always; we are peaceful. But in reality, it
doesn't seem to be so. I am unhappy, I am anxious, I am worried,
I am disturbed. That's like writing "sugar" on a piece of paper and
putting it in your hands. You can't drop that "sugar" in your coffee.
Yes, the books that you read might be books of knowledge, or you
might hear the knowledge spoken, but to really know what is being
expressed, you have to realize it. You have to experience that. And
again, to experience that, you should see it face to face. To see your
own true nature clearly, as you see your own face, you should have
a reflector or a mirror. And what is the true reflector of the soul?
Your own mind. Your own mind is there as the true mirror of the
soul. And when can you see your face well in a mirror? When the
mirror is clean and straight. If the mirror is dirty and distorted,
your face will look ugly, not because your face is truly ugly, but
because the unclear mirror reflects a distorted image; the mistake
is in the mirror. Do you get the point? Either you try to correct the
mirror, or you can change the mirror. In the same way, when you
don't see your own true happiness reflected in the mind, it's not
that you don't have happiness; it's that your mind is not fit to reflect
your happiness well. Why? Because the mind is colored or covered
or distorted. That is why Yoga asks you to keep the mind clean.

As a matter of fact, all religions ask the same thing, that you
keep the mind clean, pure. In fact, Yoga is not anything different
from religion. Yoga talks about the fundamental principles of all
the religions. In that sense, it is the basic part of every religion. It is
the religion. What you call "religion" expresses the basic principles
of the religion, not its superficial structures. What would you call

a church? You wouldn't call it a construction. If you always say, "A church must be like this," then, in this modern day, you will never see a church, right? You have all kinds of architects, so it's not the design of the building that makes the church; rather, it's the *sanctum sanctorum*. That is to say, it's the main symbol, or the altar, that makes the church. I'm just giving you a superficial example, because even the altar doesn't make the church. What makes the church a church is that divinity that you see there, that you feel there. That's what makes the church. Otherwise, even a church can be a business place. So, it's the essence in it that makes it truly a church, and that is why we say that Yoga goes to the very essence, to the essential part of every religion.

Yoga is not a religion by itself. It just ignores the superficial structures. It talks about what is inside a church, inside a synagogue, inside a temple. It talks about what makes these places sacred. In that sense, Yoga goes to the very root of your true Self. And every essential part of religion says, "Keep your mind calm and clean." There's the beautiful saying in the Bible: "Blessed are the pure in the heart; they shall see God." What does that mean? In the yogic interpretation, I may just add a couple of words to make the meaning more understandable. We would say, "Blessed are those who keep their mind calm and clean; *they shall see themselves as God*." Why? Because their true nature is God. They are the image of God. The scriptures say that God made man in His own image. As such, you are all the images of God. Part of God. Nothing less than that. And again, when will you see yourself as that God? Only when your mirror is clean. And what is your mirror? Your mirror is the mind. So keep the mind free from any coloring or covering or distortion. That is essential.

Now the questions are: What color is the mind? What gives color to the mind? What covers the mind? What distorts the mind? The basic, the very root cause for all this coloring, covering or distortion is the ego feeling: "Mine; that's mine. I must have it. Mine must be the best. I must have everything for me. I must be the topmost person." The "I" and "mine" feeling is based on the ego sense. It is that feeling that causes all calamities. You can reflect on this point. Then, you will know why you face difficulties in life. It is that "I" selfish feeling. In fact, all crimes are committed because of this attitude that "I must have that." And this attitude may not be only connected to the individual. Collectively, we may feel: "*My* community must have that. *My* family must have that. *My* country must have that." Just as two individuals fight, two countries fight. "My country must be the superpower. Therefore, don't allow any other country to win the arms race." What is the difference between the arms race of two countries and the arms race of two individuals? Essentially, none. Two people punch each other. That's also an arms race, is it not? They use their arms, maybe 24 inches of their arm. So, it is egoism, the selfishness of the individuals, is it not? The "I" and the "mine."

Therefore, again, every religion says, "Get rid of this selfishness. Be a selfless person, a dedicated person. Think of others, not yourself, first." And that is where service and sacrifice come in. When you see the Cross, what do you read from that, what is its meaning? What is the symbolic significance of the cross? It's *sacrifice*. Why do people adore the Lord Jesus Christ? Because of his great sacrifice. He didn't live for himself. He was totally selfless. So, he remains in the Self of everybody. Thus, he wins the whole world. On the other hand, a selfish person always gets into trouble. With selfishness we try to win over the world, win over the country, but Jesus never even had a sword in his hand, not to mention your machine guns and bombs. He never even had a small penknife in his hand. He just walked emptyhanded and he won the whole globe. Wherever you go, you hear people talking about the greatness of Jesus Christ, the greatness of Prophet Muhammad, the greatness of the Buddha, the greatness of Mahatma Gandhi. All those great sages and saints, they won the heart of every person without even a penknife. But here we are, trying to win a neighboring country with our atomic bombs. Still, we fail. So, what type of war do you want to win? We can be victorious, certainly, but without making any enemies.

To sum up, I want you to remember the following three points. First of all, you are the image of God, nothing less then that. If you know that right away and realize that, then you don't need to worry about anything. Wherever you are, you are beautiful, you are all corrected. Even if you remain in the correctional institution, you don't need to worry. You can think, "Wherever I am, I am wonderful."

The second point is that you keep the mind serene under all conditions. Let nothing disturb you. Certainly, nothing can disturb you if you are strong. Even a storm cannot blow out the lamp if it becomes a hurricane lamp, is it not? But take away the protection and even a breeze will blow it out. A candle that is put in the right place can face a hurricane. So, protect your mind with the spirit of dedication, with selflessness, and nobody on this earth will be able to disturb you.

If you don't live selflessly, in the spirit of dedication, then even the very religion you practice, even the very name "God" that you utter will disturb you. Haven't you seen people killing each other in the name of God, in the name of religion? Can you say that there is God, then? If a religion is going to allow you to kill each other, can you call that a religion, then? That's not really God's religion. That's humanity's egoistic religion. In the Western hemisphere and in the Eastern hemisphere, everywhere we see religious quarrels. Yet, they all say, "Love thy neighbor as thy own self." They read that in the chapel; then, they walk out with a machine gun. What's more, there are even fights between churches–"My church, my church." It is not God's church.

Whether it's the name of the race or the religion or the country or the color, how shallow we are in our thinking. Because someone's color is a little black, you say, "He is different. I am white; this is different." How far are you white? And how deep are you black, sir? Not even half a millimeter. Just scratch the skin a little; there is neither white nor black, but only red. How shallowminded we are. Just by seeing the color, we divide ourselves. When we become that superficial, we fight, we kill each other, we die. We don't go deep into that essence. Going into the essence and realizing that Oneness is what you call Yoga. Yoga means coming together, oneness.

To repeat, the dilemma is egoism. *I. Mine. My* church must build up all its members. *My* country must be the superpower. *My* race must be the dominating, ruling race. The problem is the little "i." Now I am not talking about the big, capital "I." The capital "I" is the real you, the true Self. So, free that true Self, the true, clean mind from getting contaminated. Correct the mind; keep it free. That's Yoga. And do it by any means; it doesn't matter. Do it in any name, with any label. All you have to do is undo what you have done to discolor, to disturb your mind. You don't need to do anything afterwards. All you have to do is to undo things. Once you have undone everything, you don't need to do anything; you just be. Like the fruit, like the flower, just be.

I say, again, we are all made in the image of God. Even those who worship God in an image or in a person say that God is omnipresent, omniscient. If that is so, then, God cannot be in one form. So, in that sense, God has no form, no name and that's why God is everywhere. Even the gender "He" is often used because you have to say something. God can be "He" or "She" or "It." God need not always be the Father in Heaven. God can be Mother on Earth. Or God can be an It, because everything has that consciousness. Even an atom has consciousness, is it not so? There is consciousness within an atom. The electrons have consciousness, and the nucleus has it. The nucleus sits right in the middle, watching the electron running around, like a nice, beautiful girl sitting in the middle and all the boys running around her. If they don't have consciousness, how can they make that love? This analogy illustrates that we have consciousness everywhere.

Furthermore, that omnipresent, cosmic consciousness is what you call God, and that is always serene and peaceful. But the question is: how are you going to see it, to recognize it? To know the omnipresent, formless and nameless, you should also become formless and nameless. However, as long as you are within a form and a name, you cannot grasp the formless and nameless One. You need a certain form and name. Because of your limited understanding, you bring the unlimited One to a limited level so that you can understand it. Say, for example, that I'm sitting here and

I want to know the entire country. So, I ask you, "Where is Texas? Where is Tennessee? Where is Chicago? Where is New York?" I am asking you, and what do you do? You just bring a piece of paper with lots of lines and say, "Here is New York, here is Tennessee, here is the Missouri River, and here is the Mississippi River–if you touch it, you won't get wet." So, if you want to see the place, you get to know where it is and you go there.

It's the same thing if you want to know God. God is a symbol, a symbol that reminds you to be a dedicated person. But you won't be a dedicated person just by carrying a cross, which might be an unnecessary weight on your neck. You need not carry the cross, itself, if you carry the message of the cross. But if you still want to carry the cross, fine; go ahead. However, without the message, carrying a cross is an unnecessary burden. So that means that all these symbols are aids.

To give another example, suppose I go to your room and you show me a picture, telling me, "This is my papa and mama." Am I to believe it, or not? I'd say, "What is this you are showing me, a piece of paper?" If it's just a piece of paper, can I take it and throw it away? If I did, would you be happy? You may even give me a big, beautiful punch. You won't say, "It's just a piece of paper; it doesn't matter." Why? Because you don't see it simply as a piece of paper. To you, it represents your papa and mama. That means that it's not the thing by itself that is valued. What is valued, rather, is what it represents.

All these symbols are representatives. They represent something. Like when you give a toy elephant to a child, for instance, he or she will take the toy elephant, put it in a place, feed it with a little grass and water it. To the child, the elephant is real. When the child grows older, he or she will just laugh at the toy, thinking, "My goodness, how much time I wasted in trying to feed that." That's what. Our understanding is limited. When our understanding grows, we don't need all these symbols. But as long as we are limited, we have to see through a limited thing. Another example: the sea is unlimited, but if you want to bring a little sea into your home, you have to bring it in a bucket of water, so you limit the sea according to your container. In the same way, our minds are small. We can grasp only a little. But the more you open your mind, the more you see. Make your mind unlimited and you see the unlimited God. That's what the sages say: "Open up your mind. Don't limit yourself with one caste, one community, or one country." You fill the hole in you. The really opened-up person will not even say, "I am limited to this. I belong to India; I belong to America; I belong to this church or that church." That kind of individual would not be satisfied with that but would say, "I belong to everything, to everybody. Even a rat in a small hole is my brother or sister. I belong to that rat." Such a person would never deny anything. To that person, God is everywhere and he or she sees God in a rat, in a cat, in a tiger, in a policeman, in a thief.

The point is that until you get the cosmic vision, you will belong somewhere. But you don't have to put God in a bottle, declaring, "This is what you have to believe." The whole world talks about God in different names. It's not that everybody calls God Christ or Buddha or Muhammad. Look at Hinduism; how many hundreds of images of God exist. Yet, the *Vedantic* practitioner following the *Vedic* tradition laughs completely at the images of the gods, saying, "Why, images? No." The *Vedantic practitioner* doesn't believe in images. On the other hand, the *Siddhantic* practitioner, a *Shaivite*, or worshipper of Lord Siva, does believe in images. So what happens? They fight. It's something like a kindergarten child believing in toys. An adult doesn't believe in toys, but she forgot that she was once a kindergartener. That is the trouble.

Thus, we understand from our own levels. That's why I fully agree with you that if you don't believe in seeing God or in recognizing Him in one symbol or one name, it's fine. But to you, I would say that the peace in *you,* or the happiness in *you,* is God. Keep it up. Don't allow the happiness to be destroyed by anything. And the best way is to get out of your selfishness, because it is your selfishness that gives room for the destruction of the happiness. Nobody can destroy your happiness. The peace is you; God is in you. By disturbing the peace in you, you are not going to see God anywhere. That's why in our Integral Yoga approach we say, "You take anything as your object of meditation or your idea of meditation." This approach always says, "Keep your balance. Keep your mind calm and peaceful." And anything that will make your mind peaceful, that is your method; go ahead and do it. We don't stipulate and say, "This is the only technique that will save you, that will bring a key to heaven." No.

And what is God's likeness? What is God like? Peaceful, is it not so? If God has made you in God's likeness, then you must be that, too. How can you say that God made you in God's likeness? No, it's not the scriptures that say that. We misunderstand the scriptures. If God has created everything out of Itself, then everything must be God. And if we could never become that way, why should we even worship God? What is the purpose of worshipping God? When you go to a college or a university in order to learn a specific subject, science, for example, from a professor, if the professor says, "You can never be a professor; just be a student and learn from me," why would you want to learn from that professor? Your interest will be to become a super professor.

We are all pure. We are all the image of God. God created everything. From where? Out of what? Out of nothing. Out of nothing means that in the beginning, there was only God, nothing else. Then God created the world, but from what? In the beginning, there was nothing except God. That means that everywhere, only God existed. There was only God everywhere. Then, God started creating the world. From what? From part of God, is it not so? Then, there was no longer nothing. In the beginning everything was God. There was no nothing. My question was, "In the beginning what was there?" Before the creation, did not God exist? If you doubt that, then you cannot say that God created everything. First, you should accept that in the beginning, God was. When you say, "In the beginning," do you accept that in the beginning there was God? And is there anything except God or only God? What was there? Only God, is that not so? Where was God? Everywhere? Not here? It's just a matter of understanding, that's what.

Furthermore, if you say that in the beginning there was nothing except God, only God, then there was not even heaven. You can't say that God was in heaven. There was not even heaven. There was only God, everywhere. That's why we say it's not that God created the world out of something like a carpenter created all these things out of wood, but God created everything out of Itself. That means God became the whole world. That is why we say God is present everywhere. When you create a bench, there must be the wood. God became the earth. God did not create it. Creation means that God became Itself. Say you go to the sea. You see the waves; you see the sea. Where does a wave come from? And what happens to the wave afterwards? And what is the object that you call "wave"? The wave is water, is it not? So in the sea there is nothing but water. When the water takes different shapes, then you say, "That is a wave; this is ice." In essence they are all nothing but water.

Similarly, there is only God. God appears as waves, as foam, as bubbles, as icebergs, as you, as me, as this and that, as everything. That's why the same scriptures say, God is omnipresent. What is omnipresent? God is present everywhere, as everything, not *in* everything. If God is present *in* everything, then the thing that God was in is not God. If air is in the pot, the pot is not air. Then, you cannot say air is everywhere. Air is not in the pot. So instead, we say that the air, itself, became a pot and that it is inside, outside and the pot also. So air is everywhere. And tell me, where is the atom? Is it inside something? It's everything. You are a bunch of atoms. I am also a bunch of atoms. And in between space, this is also atoms. So we are all atoms. Atoms or Adams? That's why God created Adam first. And Adam, itself, is part of two: Adam and Eve. Eve is created out of Adam, is it not so? In the same way, the electron is a part of the atom. The electron, more or less, got separated from the neutron and it runs around taming the atom.

Yes, religion is a science. In fact, science helps us to understand religion better. If you go a little deeper into the Hindu philosophy, Hindus have a symbol called *Sivalinga*. *Sivalinga* is just a kind of eggshaped stone placed on a round ring, a ring stone, so it can remain in place. Unfortunately, though, some of the Western authors interpreted the *Sivalinga* literally as the male and female organs (because even the Eastern scriptures talk in that language). The round thing is the female and the globe thing is the male and they are put together. So, the *Sivalinga* represents nothing but sexual union. But this is the wrong interpretation.

The *Sivalinga* symbolizes the atom. It symbolizes the most minute molecule of the atoms. If you view an atom properly, through a proper microscope, you will see the nucleus part jumping up and down and the electrons running around. The electron part of the atom is the negative charge, called the *feminine* charge. The positive charge that jumps up and down is the *masculine* part, the positive. If you see the coloring of the atom, the jumping up and down, the central part, you'll see that it is reddish in color. The electrons that run around give a bluish or greenish glow. If you read the Hindu scriptures, you will learn that the middle part of the *Sivalinga* is red and the round part is green. It's nothing but a symbol of the atom. That means the first manifestation of the unmanifested One.

Even that is not the very first manifestation, because there is a symbol to see. It has developed into a kind of matter, but even before that, the circular expression of the unexpressed energy, or God, is the sound. Hindu scriptures say that the first expression of God is sound. If you read the Bible, that also says, "In the beginning there was the Word." What is the Word? The Word is Sound. The Word was with God. Anything that is static when it begins to move creates sound, even a machine. Start a machine and it hums immediately. A dynamo, when you start it, it hums. That hum is the first sound. So the entire cosmos expressed as the hum, as the Word or the Sound; this is agreed upon by every scripture. Then, the sound became more clear and more dense in order to produce forms. That's why, nowadays, you can even photograph words, sound vibrations–because they are nothing but subtle matter. Therefore, matter is nothing but sound energy.

So present-day science really makes us understand religion better. And all these dogmas and practices, all these churches, synagogues, mosques and temples are aids for us to go to the very depth of our being to realize the Truth. We need all that. You may say that when two people sit and meditate, it becomes a church. Yes; I agree. Then why should we need a church? It is to create an environment. If two people can sit by themselves and meditate well, then they don't need a church. But not everybody can do that. If two people go and sit there, they won't meditate on anything. They will be gossiping. But when they come into a church, they will easily fall into the atmosphere. It helps them to meditate. It's group psychology.

Moreover, every place has its own vibrations. If you go into a laughing room, you will laugh. If you go into a crying room, you can't laugh. If you go into a hospital, you can't just whistle, jump and dance. You become a little sad. Why? Because the entire atmosphere of the hospital is like that. When you come into an institution like this, somehow you feel a little tightened, reserved. When you go to a carnival, you are totally different. Why? It has to do with the atmosphere of the area. Likewise, when you walk into a chapel, you immediately feel, "This is God's place." It reminds you; it helps you to get into that mood quickly. That is why we need a church. But if you can produce that feeling even in your home, then you don't need a church. You can be a private student; without being in the university, you can appear just for the exam. It's not that everybody should go to university.

That is the purpose behind all these institutions, spiritual and religious institutions and even gatherings. Take, for example, all these students wearing yellow. What does it mean? It's not that just by wearing yellow, they become any different. These clothes serve to remind them that they have a goal in life. They're aids. So the dress alone doesn't make a clergyman a clergyman or a doctor a doctor. Otherwise, everybody could put on a stethoscope and become a doctor. But they are symbols; they remind us; they help us. That's why we need all these things. But we shouldn't get tied up in all that. That's where sometimes we make mistakes. If somebody says, "I am a doctor," but if you don't see a stethoscope around his neck, you don't recognize him as a doctor. That's your mistake then. Spiritual symbols are also like that. If you don't wear a cross, "You are not a Catholic." The minute you wear a cross, even if you don't believe in God, you are a Catholic. That means we put stress on the symbols and not on the qualities. The symbols are to remind us. And that goes with everything in life.

You are all so wonderful. I am so happy that I came today. Before we disperse, why don't we do a little chant. *OM Shanti. OM Shanti. OM Shanti OM.* I'm sure you all know the meaning of *Shanti. Shanti* means peace. And I repeat this in *Sanskrit* because it gives a beautiful depth of vibration. Instead of "*OM*, peace, *OM* peace," it sounds like peace. So, I would really want you all to sing so that you can feel the vibration, and, toward the end, we observe one complete minute of silence. May God lead us from the unreal to the real, from the darkness of ignorance to the light of wisdom, from the fear of death to the abode of immortality. *OM* peace, peace, peace be unto all. *OM Shanti.* Thank you. Thank you.

In the Lone Star State

Satya Greenstone has been practicing and teaching Integral Yoga for a long time. In October of 1977, she and her husband, Sadasiva, joined the first staff of the brand new Yogaville Vidyalayam (Temple of Learning), the school at Yogaville East in Connecticut. In the early 70s, Satya had been teaching Integral Yoga in California, where she taught a few times in a maximum security prison; mainly, though, Satya taught Yoga in Dallas, Texas. In fact, for several years she taught in a federal minimum security prison there that was blessed with a progressive, open-minded warden who was trying a new work/release program. In this facility, prisoners were able to go in and out of the prison, and their wives and children were able to stay in the prison, making the atmosphere in this facility somewhat family-like.

The male and female prisoners wanted to practice Yoga, and Satya started teaching there once a week. After awhile, prison officials saw such improvement in the behavior of the prisoners who were taking Yoga classes that they asked Satya to increase her classes from once a week to five times a week. In fact, the behavior of these inmates had changed so much for the better that they were granted permission to go to a five-day silent Yoga retreat with Gurudev and many other retreatants. The program enjoyed enormous success, as the following anecdotes illustrates.

During the time that Satya saw the positive effects that Yoga had on the prisoners in this facility, there was one inmate who was so hostile that prison officials felt he would never be rehabilitated. Outside of prison, he'd been a hit-man. He had served in Vietnam, and he said that the government had trained him to kill. So, when he got out of the service, he hired himself out as a killer and was, subsequently, arrested and imprisoned. Somehow, this inmate felt moved to join the Yoga program. In time, he became completely transformed. He felt that only Yoga answered his questions. He had believed that his punishment was unjust; but when he learned about the theory of *karma*, he realized that he was paying off his *karmic* debt. What's more, when the assistant warden saw the incredible change in this inmate, he, himself, began attending Yoga class. Gurudev gave *satsangs (spiritual discourses)* at the prison, and when he went to Dallas to give *mantra* initiation, often some prisoners would be released to receive initiation from Gurudev.

Satya also recalled that, once, some prisoners were even allowed to go to a picnic at the home of Dr. and Mrs. Edwin Ornish, the parents of Dr. Dean Ornish, whose famous program to reverse heart disease was inspired by, and based on, Gurudev's Integral Yoga teachings. It was during this occasion, in fact, that Dr. Ornish first met Gurudev. In talks and interviews, Dr. Ornish often describes how Gurudev helped him turn his own life around during a very dark period in his life when he was a young medical student.

Of course, the success of Satya's prison Yoga program depended not only on the teacher and the students, but also on the warden, whose focus was on rehabilitation and whose insight allowed prisoners to experience the transformative effects of Yoga. In fact, when he was getting ready to retire, the warden decided to write a book about his theory of prison management. Sadly, when the time did come for the warden to retire, government officials relocated to different prisons each and every member of his staff who was trained to facilitate the Yoga program. Even the chaplain who was involved was transferred to a desk job. Never again was the program offered.

The following talk, given in July of 1976, is a sample of one of Gurudev's Dallas *satsangs*.

Dallas County Detention Center,

Dallas, Texas, July 20, 1976

To Err is Human

Beloved friends, first of all, let me thank you for giving me this opportunity to serve you in my own humble way.

I know that it's not really a pleasant thing to be in jail or in prison. But somehow, in some part of our life, we face such situations. And if we know that the purpose of the very life itself is for our continuous learning, then we accept every situation in order to learn more and to improve our own lives. It's not in colleges and universities that we learn. We learn in the very world in which we live. Every day, every minute we learn.

Life serves to give us experiences so that we can grow, and jail is also a part of these experiences. It all depends upon how you look at it. That is, if some of our actions are not desirable to the community, we are allowed to realize that and to learn better ways. Prisons and jails are not there simply to crush or to punish people. Prisons and jails exist to educate people about how to lead a better social life. And don't think that you are the only people whom destiny brought into a place like this because you have committed some crimes. Actually, there are many who do commit crimes, yet they don't come into a place like this. But these people find their own jail somewhere else. To err is human. We all make mistakes. We all commit crimes in one way or another, simple crimes or big ones. And, in a way, it is by making mistakes that we learn more.

Therefore, one should not feel bad about having committed a mistake, a crime; but a sensible, intelligent person will learn a good lesson and he or she will not repeat that mistake. That's the only difference. A fool will keep on repeating the same mistake, again and again, hundreds of times and learns the lesson in a hard way. So, jail is a place where we get an opportunity to sit quietly and think, "What happened to me? Why am I here? What went wrong?" We should take this experience as an opportunity to go within, to analyze our own motivation and then to change it. In fact, you can think of prison as a sort of spiritual place–an *ashram*, as we call it—where you reform yourself; and the techniques that are given in the name of Yoga are very helpful to clean your mind and your body, so that you can help to clean your society.

Cleanliness comes from within, so only clean people will have a clean society. Many a time, we see people wanting to reform others without thinking of reforming themselves. We want to be clean all over, but these types of people don't want to become clean within first. That is to say that whatever you want to happen outside, should happen within you first. Without that, even if there is peace, you won't be able to recognize it. To know that there is peace outside, you should have peace inside. Thus, self-correction, self-reformation is very important, and we should treat places like this for that purpose. We should feel, "Yes; I am getting an opportunity."

Furthermore, you should not even see the authorities as dictatorial, dominating people who are ready to crush you or punish you. No. Treat these people as educators. And they should also treat you as students who have come here to learn more. Then, this facility becomes a beautiful place. It's all in the mind. If you treat this place as a punishing place, a jail, it's a jail. However, if you treat this facility as a meditative place, as a place where you have the opportunity to meditate, then it becomes a place of meditation. Take people who go to hospitals. Why do they go to the hospital? They go to get cured of their ailments. Similarly, this place is another form of hospital, where people go to be cured of diseases. What's more, diseases are not always physical; there are mental diseases also. It's a diseased mind that commits mistakes, so that also needs to be treated. And nobody should be condemned for his or her mistakes. Sometimes, in fact, the people who condemn others because of their mistakes would, themselves, have made the same mistakes before. It would be like a fast-running Olympic champion laughing at a little baby who crawls, forgetting that she, the champion, was also a baby once. We all went through that. If I am sitting here talking to you now, probably before, I would have sat there, listening to somebody talking to me. Today's sinner could be tomorrow's saint and today's saint could be yesterday's sinner.

Thus, we should not discourage or condemn anybody. Instead, we should always think that we are learning more and more and more. And one way of learning is by accepting whatever comes in life. If you want to clean up your life, just remember the following analogy. Think of a small shirt that wants to get cleaned because it's dirty. The shirt won't want to be pampered. You can't just simply fold the shirt and keep it on the shelf and expect it to get cleaned. It has to get drenched and suffocated in water, it has to get saturated with detergents and it has to get boiled in water. In other words, the shirt has to undergo a certain type of suffering. But the purpose of the suffering is to make the material, the shirt, clean. Likewise, the mind goes through a cleansing process.

Pain, Pain, Pain Means Gain, Gain, Gain

Sometimes, we go through suffering. The scriptures say: "Blessed are the sufferers." Why? Because it is only through suffering that we get cleaned, not by pampering. Nothing gets better by simply pampering.

Take a rock, for example. For a crude rock to have become a beautiful statue, that rock has had to have undergone a lot of suffering, a lot of hits by the hands of the sculptor. Life is like that. And if you accept it, if you accept the suffering as a way of cleaning yourselves, then you are free from so much hatred and animosity. If you don't accept it, then you are like a little baby. The baby doesn't want to accept the mother giving it a bath, so it revolts, it shouts, it wants to jump out of the bath. But the mother knows: "Unless I do it, I can't clean the baby." When you grow up, though, you accept that you need a bath to get clean. So, it's a matter of accepting.

In simple words, I say, "Pain, pain, pain means gain, gain, gain. No pain, no gain." Remember that always. I'm not saying this only here, in this correctional facility. I say this everywhere, because the whole world is a form of jail. Only through pain, do we gain much–not through pleasure. There, people need not always look for pleasure. Rather, they should look for pain.

To give another example: Dig a small hole, put a seed inside it and close up the hole. How painful it is for the seed. The seed is jailed, imprisoned. But the seed accepts it and it undergoes a lot of pain to break the earth and come up with two leaves. And unless that is done, the seed won't grow into a beautiful plant or into a big tree that will produce thousands of fruits for people. That's life. Without hardship, without suffering, we will not grow. So don't always look for pleasure, whether it is inside the jail or outside. People who look forward to pleasure really get disappointed quite a lot. Most anxieties, worries and psychotic cases develop because people expect a lot: "I just want this and that!" When they don't get what they want, they go crazy.

Thus, life should be understood well. That's the only way to grow. And that's a part of the yogic thinking. I know, you've probably heard more about *Hatha Yoga*—you might be doing some *asana*s and *pranayama*—and my introduction seems to be totally different from what you heard or what you even expected from my talk. You might have expected that the Swami was going to say, "Stand on your head for a few minutes more and you'll be all right." Let your teachers do that. I'm not here to say the same thing again. I want you to stand on your feet more than on your head. That's part of Yoga. You should learn to stand well on your own feet. Even if you don't do the headstand, it doesn't matter, because Yoga makes for a clean life, physically and mentally and, thus, a clean society, a clean environment.

Raising above Man-Made Distinctions

In addition, it doesn't matter what you are, who you are. Don't see people in relation to their color, caste, community, race, religion. No. That's all very superficial. It's your character that's important—how good you are, how clean your mind is, how universal your outlook is. That's part of Yoga: coming together, seeing everybody as one's self, seeing thyself in your own neighbor. That's Yoga. So we have to raise ourselves above all these man-made distinctions.

Of course, there are natural differences, but those differences are superficial. If a white man lives in India for a few years, he becomes black or brown. If you go to live in Alaska, you'll probably become white. Weather conditions, climactic conditions, languages; where you live, you speak that language. We should raise above all these differences. Differences are for our fun, for our happiness. But, essentially, we are all the same in spirit. The divine spirit that is in you, in me, in her, in him, it is all the same. God made human beings in God's own image, we say. I go one step further and say not only human beings. God made everything in God's own image. Even an atom is made God's image. A plant, a worm, everything is God's image.

There is a divine essence in everything and it's in that essence that we come together. We can never come together by seeing the unity in body and mind. Bodies vary, minds vary. There are no two individuals who have similar minds, a hundred per cent. No. Taste differs. Accept that. If that is your taste, okay; this is my taste, okay. But we both have the same spirit. Similarly, *what* you eat is immaterial. It's *why* you eat that is important. Suppose I ask you why you eat, will there be any differences in the answers that come from a white man or a black man or a fool or an illiterate or an intelligent man? They all give the same answer, is it not? But if I ask you what you eat, then, certainly, there will be lots of differences. You may like bread, the other person may like pudding and the third person may like spaghetti. It doesn't matter what you eat. What matters is that you all eat for the same purpose. And it's the same throughout life. There are many examples. It may be the difference in our color, the difference in the language we speak, or the difference in the way we worship. However, we should always think in terms of spiritual unity; then, we become what is called a "clean person." A clean person will not limit him- or herself to these differences. If you are a clean person, you rise above all the differences, you transcend all these limitations, you rise above all the man-made differences and you recognize the God-made unity. It is for that sake that we are given these experiences, which are really good opportunities for us to think well.

I hear, sometimes, that you complain that you don't even have windows to see outside. You have seen enough outside. Take the opportunity to see within you. That is the best thing to see. Don't try to be always extroverted. When you go into a shrine room, you close your eyes to think of God; you don't see anything outside. How many people spend thousands of dollars and go all the way to Jerusalem to stand in front of the beautiful altar and, then, to close their eyes. Why? Because the real God is not really outside; it is inside. So in a way, your experience here is helping you to look within. I would love to be here, because there's so much protection. Here, nobody will come to disturb me if I decide to sit and meditate. But outside, I may have many disturbances. Think that this is a place of meditation for you. Your entire outlook will be different.

In fact, if all the people who are incarcerated in this jail think of it as a meditation place, then they will make this jail a meditation center. Thus, it's the way that you look at it. That is, you change your vision. See the experience in the proper light and make use of it for your benefit instead of developing a sort of dislike or hatred. Those kinds of feelings will never, never help us grow. They will actually make our existence, our environment worse. And remember, nobody is going to be here eternally. So, that is the Yogic thinking.

I think at this point, I should invite you to ask questions.

Inner Peace through Meditation

Question: I was reading a book called Satan is Alive on Planet Earth, *and it said that through meditation, Yoga, and some of the other disciplines, you are opening yourself up to the occult, to Satanism and you are letting the evil forces in. Will you comment on that?*

Sri Gurudev: Well, it is because it is you who project the whole world outside. As you think, so you become. Change your thinking and you have changed the whole world. A thief will not have confidence in anyone else. A thief will see everybody as a thief. An innocent baby looks at everybody as innocent. And why does the baby see everyone as innocent? The baby sees everybody as innocent because the baby's mind is an innocent mind. That's what. It's a matter of changing our attitude. And meditation helps us to change our attitude, to change our thinking, to reform ourselves. Once you have reformed yourself, you have reformed the whole world. Work within yourself first.

We all know that the big thinkers, the great thinkers, the so-called political leaders and others talk a lot about peace, is it not so? You all know that. The world has seen many a peace talk in many big places. Have you ever seen any peace, anywhere, coming out of any of those talks? They haven't achieved anything. In fact, things seem to be getting worse and worse. Why? There's no peace because the participants go to talk about peace without having peace in themselves. Or you begin a peace march to Washington and it ends up as a riot. Why? You don't have peace. If you have peace, you don't need to march. So, if ever you want to see anything happen outside, see that it happens within you first. That's the benefit of meditation. You know yourself. And then, you don't even need to talk about peace; you simply walk as a peaceful person and people recognize that.

On this subject, I always give a little analogy. A number of unlit candles came together for a conference, and the theme was light. All the unlit candles had a long argument about how to get light, but there was total darkness in the room. Finally, one candle got really tired of the whole show, walked out and saw a lit candle somewhere in a corner. It went over and spoke to that candle, got a little spark from that candle and then, walked into the conference hall–there was light. The candle didn't even say, "Hey; I am giving you light!" It came lit. And everybody recognized it.

In other words, you don't need to go and say, "Hey, I am going to give you peace!" No. You simply go there and everyone will recognize whether you are a peaceful person or not. It's not something that you talk about. You live that life. If a happy person walks in, everybody will know: "Oh, he is happy or she is happy." You can't say, though, while you are crying, "Oh, I am happy." No. You just live that life. And that develops only through meditation. Take time to think of yourself. Develop within you the quality that you want to see outside of you. It's like photography. Whatever you want to see in the film, you have to capture inside first and then project it. Our mind is like photographic film. You capture certain qualities within you, you develop them within you and then you project your own world outside.

So, meditation is very important. Wherever you are, you should take a little time, both in the morning and in the evening to sit quietly, to think about yourself, to ask, "How am I?" "What is wrong with me?" Don't always try to find the mistakes outside. Ask, "What is wrong with me?" And correct it. Then, you will see friends and friends only everywhere. That's the beauty of meditation. Thank you for asking this question.

Yoga Psychology

Question: Is Yoga a form of self-employed psychology?
Sri Gurudev: Yes, you can say so. Yes, because Yoga deals completely with the mind. Well, why Yoga? Even religion is a form of psychology. Every religion teaches how to build up good thoughts in the mind and how to get rid of selfishness, which creates all the problems. The worst thing with the mind is its fixation with I, me, mine! That's the worst thing. So the scriptures teach us: don't put your self forward; put God forward; put humanity forward–you, thee, thou. Thus, all religion is a form of psychology.

Of course, religions express their facts in a sort of indirect way. However, in Yoga we don't particularly prescribe certain forms or rituals or this or that, because it's universal. Yoga is accepted by people whether they are Catholic, Protestant, Jewish, Muslim, Buddhist, or Hindu; it's accepted by everybody. Yoga offers scientific facts about the mind, asking: How does the mind function? And when the mind is disturbed, Yoga asks: Why? What is the reason? What was the attitude with which the mind was functioning to make it disturbed? In simple language, I can say why people go to psychiatrists. People go to psychiatrists because they get frustrated. This means that they experience a lot of disappointments in their lives and they try to find somebody to use as an excuse for their disappointment. But what I say is that it is *you*. You are the cause of your disappointment, since you made an *appointment* and your own appointment got *dis-ed*. And you call it *disappointment*. If you had not made an appointment, would you have dis-appointment?

It's all about selfish appointments: *I want to grab something. I want to get something.* Then if you don't get it, you are disappointed and you blame somebody else for that. It's psychology. Yoga is a beautiful form of psychology. And in this Yoga psychology, you don't always need to depend on a psychiatrist or a psychologist. You become the psychologist for yourself. You take your mind, put it out there and question it: "Hey, what are you?" That's what you call meditation. You talk to your own mind. "What happened to you? Why this disappointment? Oh, I know; you made that appointment. Therefore, if you don't want disappointment, don't make appointments." You tell this to your own mind. You become the doctor for your mind. The mind becomes the patient. So, you don't always have to pay $25 for half an hour. No. This process is called *self-reformation*.

Of course, in this form of psychology, you also believe in a higher power, a higher consciousness. "Higher" here refers to the cosmic, that is, the cosmic consciousness, a part of which is functioning in you–others may call that *God*. In other words, you believe in something higher. You can receive that higher consciousness. You can communicate with it. You can tune your heart to receive it. That is probably the only difference between Western psychology and Yoga psychology. That is, Yoga psychology says that because mind has its own limitations, with our limited mind it is even hard to understand the unlimited one. So, the only way to understand the unlimited is to link your limited mind with the unlimited. It's like a drop of water in the sea trying to understand the sea. The drop can't step outside the sea to know the sea. That's why the scriptures say: "I am thine. All is thine. Thy will be done." You unite your littleness to that vast One.

The Purpose of Yoga

Question: How long have you been practicing Yoga? When one starts to practice Yoga, which is preferable: to start first with Hatha Yoga or to seek first to clear the mind? What would be the proper food to eat in order to stabilize oneself?

Gurudev: These are beautiful questions. Before I answer them, we should know why we want to practice Yoga. We should know the purpose of it. The purpose of practicing Yoga is to keep a sound body and a sound mind. Remember that: we practice Yoga to be physically and mentally sound. That is the aim behind all these practices. If that is so, then, we should think, "What makes the body and mind unsound?" And we should stay away from whatever that may be. That's all.

I should also say that you cannot *make* the mind peaceful. Simply, if you leave the mind undisturbed, then it's peaceful. To understand this idea, imagine that you have a bowl of water. What would you do to make the water peaceful? You wouldn't do anything. You wouldn't disturb it, is it not so? Then it is peaceful. In the same way, the body and mind, by nature, are peaceful. That's why even the very term disease should be questioned. What do you mean by "disease?" You have disturbed your "ease." Am I right? You had "ease" before and you disturbed it, so you are "diseased." Thus, even to fall into disease, you should have had ease before. So, ease is your nature. Peace is your nature. Stay away from disturbing it.

If this teaching is well understood, then you know the importance of *Hatha Yoga*, proper food, meditation, everything. You know that they all help you in not disturbing your ease. Food, for example, is an important factor, both in relation to our body and to our mind in order to maintain the soundness of the physical and mental aspects of our being. With proper food, you have proper health. But if you eat a lot of junk food, you'll find that this leaves a lot of toxins in the system, giving room for all sorts of problems. All types of rheumatism, kidney problems, cancer and this and that are due mainly to eating the wrong foods. We seem to blame the little, unseen viruses that are here and there. No. It's wrong food. And food not only affects the body, but it affects the mind as well. In fact, if anybody wants to see clearly how the body and the mind are affected by food, then I would recommend them to go to the zoo.

Yes, go to the zoo to see all the animals and look at what they eat. You'll see that all the animals that are caged, that are foul smelling and that are mentally restless, eat one kind of food. And you'll see that the animals that are left alone, those that are walking gently, looking at you, smilingly with no foul smell—even if you poke your nose into a goat's mouth, you won't experience a foul smell—eat a different kind of food.

And it's not just animals. People are also like that. Some are afraid of even raising their arms, because . . . [Gurudev makes a gesture to indicate a foul smell]. But people hide the bad odor with . . . [Gurudev imitates someone spraying himself with underarm deodorant]. Why? Why does all that junk come out through their perspiration? It comes out because they put all those things into themselves. However, if you are a strict vegetarian, you don't need to be afraid of all these offensive odors. You don't need deodorant. So, food is very important.

People think: "Oh, this is just religion. No. But, after all, what is religion? Religion is to help you live a sound life, to help you experience nice, healthy living. You become physically and mentally pure. You see God. That is the reason why, even in so-called different religious groups, where people normally eat all kinds of food, members refrain from eating all that on auspicious days. On Easter Sunday, for instance, nobody eats the wrong food. Why? Because people want to call that a holy day; isn't that so? Therefore, you make it a holy day by not eating the wrong food. But if you don't eat the wrong food throughout your life, then your entire life becomes a holy life. So food is very important.

Of course, we don't insist in the beginning that you give up all the unhealthy food. Let people realize the importance of it themselves. We simply suggest that–if possible–you stay away from the wrong food. Stay away from smoking. Stay away from liquor. With regard to smoking, for example, our lungs are not created for nicotine. I heard that if you are a little good here, you are given a little gift of a pack of cigarettes. Is it so? Yes? What kind of gift is that? Then, if you are good, should you be given a little poison as a gift? I really request the authorities to stop that. Give them some candy bars if you want. No cigarette gift. Gift? A cigarette is not a thing to be gifted. No. It's poison. It spoils the lungs. It pollutes the lungs. You not only want ecology outside, you want ecology inside, also. God never made the lungs to accept poison with nicotine, which creates lot of problems. We pay for our poison while nectar, that is oxygen, is free. If you decide to take a deep breath, will they be sending you a big bill at the end of the month because you inhaled a little more, extra oxygen? No. But if you decide to take an extra puff, you have to pay a little extra money. So understand that whatever will allow you to maintain your health is good for you. That's where the food and the drink and the smoking all come in.

Then, which to begin first, *Hatha Yoga* or meditation? It's according to your temperament. That is to say if you feel like doing it, good; because the body and mind work together. If one falls sick, the other will be disturbed. Therefore, it is always good to attack from both sides. To explain further, say that you try to sit and meditate for a while, but, within a couple of minutes, your ankle complains, "Oh I can't sit anymore." In this situation, what is it you are meditating on? You are meditating on your ankle, probably, not on God. So, take care of the body. Let the body be at ease first. If you sit comfortably, you should be able to forget the body. And which part of the body will you easily forget? The healthy part.

I'll ask you one question: Did you ever think of your little toe? [Someone answers: "Only if it hurts."] That's a simple, beautiful answer. Yes, only when it is sick, do you think of it. When it is not sick, you forget it. Likewise, you never think of the stomach, unless it is hungry. That's what. A diseased part will always draw your attention. You won't have time for anything else then. So it's good to take care of the body and to say to it, "Okay, now you are healthy, so don't bother me anymore. Let me do something else." *Hatha Yoga* is really very good for that. It takes away all the toxins. It helps you get out of all these habits.

Even a person who smokes a lot can benefit from the Yoga practices. If you do *pranayama* (breathing practices) regularly, you will get your lungs cleaned and you cannot even tolerate smoke anymore. I have seen people who smoked packs and packs and packs; now, they cannot even sit near somebody in a train who smokes. It's as though they were total non-smokers from birth. Why? Because they cleaned their lungs that way. Do what's right and the wrongs go away. *Hatha Yoga* is a beautiful beginning, because everybody can easily work with the body first. Then, too, the charm in doing *Hatha Yoga* is that you cannot do *Hatha Yoga* well without calming your mind. That is, *Hatha Yoga* is not some physical drill. The minute you lie down to do the Cobra Pose, you go into a meditative situation. Think of your body, think of your spine; do it slowly. Without the cooperation of the mind, you can't do it well. So indirectly the mind also is trained.

That's why, afterwards, you go slowly into the other fields of Yoga. Many thousands here in this country have gone into meditation through *Hatha Yoga*, because it's easy to handle something gross and then go into the subtle areas. But what we always teach in Integral Yoga is a little quiet sitting, maybe a little peace chant: *OM Shanti, OM Shanti, OM.* Even the way you say *OM Shanthi* helps you to find that peace. You are calmed down. Then, you do a few postures; and then you do a little breathing, because breathing calms the mind a lot. If you are really agitated, if you are going to be bursting out, suddenly sit back and take a few slow deep breaths; immediately, you calm the mind, and your anger goes away somewhere. Breath and mind go together. If your mind is agitated, your breath is agitated. You can see this very well.

For instance, if someone maybe uses a wrong word and you get disturbed, immediately watch your breath. You will be breathing vehemently. "Ahh, Ahh. That fellow said that to me!" The mind got the idea, and it affected the breath, and vice versa. Therefore, if you calm the breath, you have calmed the mind. And it is easier to calm the breath than it is to calm the mind, because the mind is much subtler than the breath. So, we do a little breathing. After that, we sit quietly again, ending with a minute or two of meditation. In meditation, you just sit. You become aware of your self. You can focus your awareness on your breath, watching the breath. Or, if you like, you can repeat some holy names, according to your own faith, or you can use OMMM. It doesn't matter which holy names, words or sounds you use. Just let the mind dwell on one thing. Then it becomes restful.

Actually, it's even good to sleep that way. Every day, before you go to bed, lie down and watch your breath or say a *mantra*. You get the best sleep, without any sleeping pills. Since Yoga started this *mantra* business, sleeping pill prices and sales have gone down. Nobody needs sleeping pills anymore. And you never get overdosed, because this is the right way of doing things. We're not putting in one poison in place of another poison.

In this regard, I've often told the drug rehabilitation programs that they can never, never help a heroin addict with methadone. It's only temporary; and instead of putting in one poison, you are putting in another poison. Now, it's a known fact that people get overdosed with methadone. They get addicted to methadone. But we have cured many, many people from heroin addiction just by breathing practices, just by *Hatha Yoga*. You put something positive into the system. You don't substitute one poison for another poison. The yogic approach is cleaner and more positive. If at any time you decide not to do Yoga, you can stay away from it for a week or two, and you don't go crazy because you're not doing the *asana*s. But if you smoke and you miss even one cigarette, you go crazy. Why? Because it's a wrong habit.

Leading a Calm Life

Questioner: How long you have been involved in Yoga?
Sri Gurudev: Oh, me? Well, somehow, from the very birth, from the very childhood. I was a little fortunate in being born into a yogic family. When I say Yoga, it need not always be *Hatha Yoga*. Of course, the *Hatha Yoga* part I started at the age of 28. But before that, we were doing meditation, prayers. That's also part of Yoga. Yoga is not necessarily only *Hatha Yoga*. My mamma would not even give me breakfast if I didn't say my prayers. Yes, that's the way we were trained. We were lucky in that way. I started *Hatha Yoga* at the age of 28. Now, though, I don't have time to do that much; but still, my body is very flexible. Even after a break of a number of years, I can still do all the *asanas*. My body is never rigid, because I take care of my food. I eat only once a day and I don't eat any solid food in the morning or in the evening. Occasionally, when I go out, if the host insists, I may take something just to satisfy him or her. Otherwise, one meal a day, that's enough for me. And I do a lot of work. I work on tractors, I chop wood, I drive; and that's enough for me. Don't think that guru means always sitting on thrones like

this. No. We work a lot in the community. How old am I? Can you guess? I knew you are going to ask that.

Answer: I would be dishonest if I didn't say that I heard you were around sixty-five.

Sri Gurudev: That's what you heard. But now after seeing me, do I look that?

Answer: No

Sri Gurudev: Only the gray beard sometimes deceives people.

Answer: I'm only thirty-seven and mine is getting gray.

Sri Gurudev: I still feel young. I feel like I'm 25. I have that much energy. A couple of months back, about 35 students came with me for a short world tour. At one point, we were climbing a mountain, walking. All these people, they couldn't follow me. I was literally running up and they were gasping, staying behind, far away. It's all due to Yoga, clean living.

More than anything else, my mind is always peaceful. I never worry about anything. I never allow my peace to be disturbed. Because I don't want things–power, position, name, fame. If they come: "Oh, you have come, okay. Let it be." When they decide to go: "Okay. Go." That's all.

People might have told you that I have established centers, 25 centers coast-to-coast. Don't trust them. I have never established any center. Students form into a group and they ask me to come and serve them. I go. I didn't even come to this country to establish any centers, wanting to be a guru. No. I never wanted anything. When people came to me, I didn't want them to feel rejected. I said, "Okay, you came; all right, stay." If they wanted to go, I said, "Do you want to go? Okay, go."

"Take it easy" is my saying. My mind never gets agitated over anything. You may praise me today; tomorrow you may blame me. There will be beautiful write-ups today; tomorrow they will say, "Oh, you rogue; you've cheated everybody." I'll say, "Fine." It's all beautiful to me. I never make appointments, so I never get disappointed. Keeping the mind peaceful is very important to staying young. Sometimes, you are physically young, but you are always worried, anxious over anything, with a lot of disappointments. That makes you become old very soon. How many 16- or 17-year-old kids look like grannies? It's because there's so much of anxiety, so much disturbance in the mind.

Lead a calm life. Trust in God. Whatever has to happen, will happen. You are not the reformer of the whole world. You didn't create the world. Keeping a cool mind is very, very important. Yes. It will take care of the body, also. Calm and cool and composed.

Samatvam yoga ucyate: Equanimity of mind is Yoga. You can always maintain that. That is what you call purity of heart. "Blessed are the pure in heart, for they shall see God," says the scripture. What is purity? Staying neutral, not taking sides, keeping your calm, that is the real secret of healthy and happy living. And it's not the monopoly of only a few people, ascetics living in the Himalayas, growing a long beard. You can do that. Everybody can do that. It's our birthright.

In fact, I really want you all to enjoy that peace. Don't worry about all this here. These are all just temporary phases, different stages, various scenes in the drama of life. They come and go. Don't think that you are really in a jail. It's just that this is the part you are playing. After all, in the whole drama of life, there are jail scenes, also. Think of it that way. Don't let your mind get affected by these things. Be nice to everybody. Don't even look at them with a sort of hard face: "Oh, these people are really going to hurt me." Treat everybody as your brother and sister. Let there be beautiful communication here. And it's possible. If you just change your mind and decide to see it that way, you will see everybody as a friend here. You'll make this place a heaven. It's possible. It's all what you make of it.

I hope that these few ideas will really help you make your life a little more peaceful, harmonious and that you will be pleased by the authorities and the authorities will be pleased by you. Just imagine that you are all helping each other. They learn a lot from you. You learn a lot from them. Yes.

I really wish you a peaceful existence. And when you come out, you'll be better and more beautiful citizens equipped to create a better world.

God bless you. Peace be with you. Thank you. *OM Shanti.*

Chapter 3
The East Coast Prison Experience

While we are free to choose our actions, we are not free to choose the consequences of our actions —Stephen R. Covey

John (Margabandhu) Martarano, director of the Integral Yoga Institute of Fairlawn, New Jersey, became involved with Gurudev and Integral Yoga in the late 1960s. An unhealthy lifestyle had left him ill, and he found that Yoga—and the raw food diet that he still follows today—could help him restore his physical and mental health. He'd also found his spiritual path.

By 1970, Margabandhu was running an Integral Yoga Center in a house in Morristown, New Jersey. A psychologist from the area who took Yoga classes at the center was working in a prison, and she asked Margabandhu to participate in a study of the effects of Yoga on the prison population (she also included biofeedback techniques in her study). He agreed and began going to Morris County Prison three or four days a week to teach meditation, *pranyanama* and *Hatha Yoga*. A grant was awarded so that both the psychologist and Margabandhu could get paid. And that was just the beginning for Margabandhu, who ended up teaching in the maximum security prison three days a week for seven or eight years. Eventually, however, the new county administrators stopped awarding the grant and the political climate changed, so even though Margabandhu offered to continue teaching without pay, the program was ended.

Sri Gurudev was invited to speak at the Morris County Prison and he did speak there several times. In fact, Margabandhu remembers one occasion very well.

Besides teaching at the prison, Margabandhu had also been teaching at Farleigh Dickinson, a local university, and Sri Gurudev was invited to speak there, too. Margabandhu had already been working at the prison for a couple of years, and some of the inmates who were on work relief found out about Gurudev's upcoming talk at the school and they wanted to go. Prison officials approved their request, provided that Margabandhu would transport them and be fully responsible for getting them back to the prison. So, on the day of the talk, Margabandhu picked up the six inmates and drove them to the university.

Sri Gurudev's talk that day was all about selfless service. And, as he often did, he spoke about cleanliness, mentioning as an example that when we use a bathroom, we should leave it cleaner than we had found it. Margabandhu got so deeply involved in what Gurudev was saying that he hadn't noticed that one of the inmates, a tough, rugged guy, was missing. After a little while, he turned to check on the men, noticing then that one man was gone. Margabandhu was beside himself, even worrying that he would have to take that prisoner's place. But after almost a half hour, the man appeared. He had gotten so inspired by what Gurudev was saying that he went out, got a mop and cleaned the university bathroom until it was spotless. Margabandhu was so touched that he started to cry.

Once, Sri Gurudev even advised prison officials to change the prison diet to a vegetarian diet, explaining that meat has a negative effect on the emotions, stimulating restless, aggressive tendencies. The authorities were so impressed that they extended the grant.

Morris County Prison also housed a section for women inmates and some of these women took Yoga classes with Margabandhu. In the summer of 1973, the students asked Margabandhu to arrange for Gurudev to visit them. A visit was organized for July 30 and the women were eager to share their thoughts and interests and to pose some questions to Gurudev about the yogic lifestyle.

Morris County Prison – Women's Section
Morris County, New Jersey, July 30, 1973

In a Strong Mind, There's No Room for Anxiety

Question: I didn't get the drop in anxiety that I expected from Yoga. It was surprising. I talked to Marg [Margabandhu] about that, and he said that you don't expect that right away.

Sri Gurudev: Well, reducing the anxiety takes a while, because the mind has to be educated. That is where Yoga need not be restricted to only the physical postures. The breathing is very important. The breathing also really takes care of the mind. The mind is greatly calmed just by the breathing.

Question: Just by the breathing?

Sri Gurudev: Yes, and even by slow breathing with concentration on the breath. For example, when you do alternate breathing, your mind should be on the breath. Even while we're doing the breathing, you can see the tension decreasing. The mind gets calm in our meditation, because we begin with slow breathing to calm the mind; then, we go into the meditation. The breathing helps a lot. And soon after the breathing, you can slowly get into a kind of gentle chanting, some *OM Shanti, OM Shanti,* a *mantra* that creates a vibration of peace, so that you can feel the peace. Then, you can simply sit quietly, observing what is happening within you. You're not doing anything. The real meditation is not to do anything; it's just to observe. That will simply loosen everything. And when the mind relaxes like that, the mind gets stronger. Anything that gets relaxed and gets rest becomes strong, and it's like that with the mind, also. When you relax the mind, it becomes gentle and slowly it becomes stronger and stronger. And in a strong mind, there is no room for any anxiety.

Question: But this all takes time.

Sri Gurudev: That's why we always include some other elements along with the physical postures. It's not just mere *Hatha Yoga* alone. That is the reason why we call our Yoga *Integral Yoga.* Integral Yoga is a combination of everything. You can even include a little discussion with your students: "What causes your anxiety?" By your own anxiety, you become more disturbed and unfit. Take a doctor, for example. A doctor can easily perform operations on other patients, but when the same doctor is going to perform surgery on his or her own spouse or child, he or she will get anxiety.

Question: So that's why there's a law against doctors operating on their own family members?

Sri Gurudev: Yes; they don't do it.

Balancing the System with a Vegetarian Diet

Staff member: We are going to try a diet without sugar for a month, because we have found that many people who have had an alcohol or drug problem just have bad eating habits or have been under stress and have the tendency to have low blood sugar. So, we're going to try a diet that will balance the system.

Sri Gurudev: Have you tried a vegetarian diet? Well, in simple language, I'll share an example that shows how different types of attitudes are related to the different types of food. Just go to the zoo. See the animals. See their attitude. All the carnivorous animals are caged, and they are restless, while the herbivorous animals are so peaceful and gentle, grazing and looking and smiling at you. Normally, the mental attitude between carnivores and herbivores is totally different. There are exceptions. Take the monkey, which is so restless, and yet, it's a vegetarian. But with the majority of animals, there's a marked difference between the carnivorous and the herbivorous animals. Another aspect is their excretion. The excreta of the carnivorous animals are terribly foul smelling, whereas with the herbivore, you don't smell anything.

Question: What about chickens?

Sri Gurudev: Chickens are not herbivorous. Furthermore, vegetarians need not use any deodorant. That's true. Their perspiration will never smell bad. We're always trying all possible ways to make ourselves a little cleaner and better looking and nice smelling. But we are only spraying away the odor. It's normal that all the foul things that we put into our systems come out of the system as foul odors, because that's what we put in. However, if you are a strict vegetarian, you don't need to use deodorant, because you don't have any perspiration odor from anywhere, whether it is from your armpit, from your face, or from anywhere. I can guarantee that. Because I've been a vegetarian from birth, I never smell. Sometimes, people even say that I smell fine, that I give off a nice fragrance. Also, you may think that if you are a vegetarian, you won't have enough strength, because you may not be getting enough protein. But that's not that case.

Question: Do you find that the food that's available in this country for people who would like to follow a vegetarian diet is generally good enough for them to be healthy?

Sri Gurudev: Are you referring to the quantity?

Question: I'm referring to the food that's available: our frozen vegetables, our leaf lettuce; we don't have too many protein vegetables available.

Sri Gurudev: You have plenty of protein in lentils and soybeans. You know, even in the case of protein, the protein that you get from the meat diet is too concentrated, and it's not free from any kind of disease-producing elements, whereas the protein that you get from lentils and other vegetables is more easily digestible. We don't need that concentrated protein. In fact, it's not that we consume all the protein and absorb it into the system. Much of it just goes out.

Question: And you do think that the vegetables and beans that our supermarkets sell are sufficient for people to be healthy?

Sri Gurudev: The vegetables and beans that we have in the supermarkets are, for the most part, not organic. But if people begin to eat organic, then the farmers will grow more organic food. In any case, eating vegetables and beans from the supermarket is still better than eating frozen meat. Last night, in Virginia, I had this same discussion. I held up a tomato and asked, "Would you want to have this tomato chemically treated? Everyone said, "No; we want organic."

Yes, you are interested in eating an organic tomato. On the other hand, *you* don't want to be organic. That is to say, how much stuff do you put into your system? Do you use drugs? Do you put all kinds of chemicals into your system? Why do you believe in drugs? Don't you want to be organic? Are you worth less than the tomato? People don't think about it, that's what. In fact, if we could just analyze our habits, in many ways we might feel ashamed. Once, a doctor who came complained that he was a heavy smoker and that he couldn't stop. He'd been smoking for the past thirty or thirty-five years. I told the doctor, "Doctor, you are a doctor. You should know anatomy. You should know what happens when some air goes into the lungs. You should know why you breathe, why you need oxygen. When you smoke, instead of putting oxygen into your body, you put nicotine into it. Do you think that you can purify your breath with nicotine or improve the lung capacity with nicotine? No wonder you complain about your heart. As he was listening to me, he became paler and paler and paler. Yes. He finally said, "All these years, I didn't think in these terms. Here I am a doctor; I know everything. But I am not practicing it for myself. I can easily administer this advice to others. Swamiji, you have opened my eyes. No more cigarettes." Immediately, he stopped smoking. His name is Dr. Obeysekere and he is now a famous heart specialist in Ceylon [Sri Lanka]. He even visits this country now and then. He is one of my students. It's only if you make people think and if they can be convinced that they will decide to quit a bad habit. The key here is that they must be convinced; they can't be forced. Force doesn't work. That's very important.

Transformation through Yoga–Even in Prison

In many cases, from listening to me speaking, violent prisoners became beautiful seekers, spiritual seekers. You help them to understand why they are in prison. You convince them that they are not forced to be here; rather, they are being treated, that it's like being in a hospital–it's for our own benefit when we spend time in a hospital.

Staff Question: We feel that many of our prisoners come here, more or less, on purpose. Many of them are not really caught by accident. They, more or less, deliberately got themselves into a certain situation. Does that fit in with your thinking about it? And what are you going to say to them about not choosing such situations?

Sri Gurudev: What is their reason for coming in deliberately? Is it just for free food and a secluded place?

Officer: They come to rely on somebody else to keep them. In other words, they come to depend on somebody else.

Sri Gurudev: That's an easy way of thinking. If that's the case, then why can't they make the best use of the situation, starting industries, for example? Let them work!

Staff Question: Do you hope that by the time the inmates leave, they'll have changed because of practicing Yoga, that they'll have become more peaceful?

Sri Gurudev: I'm not just hoping. I have hundreds of examples from different countries. Prison can often bring about a very big change in somebody's life. For instance, some of the prisoners from Ceylon [Sri Lanka] came out of prison as very peaceful individuals. They have their own temples and churches, and many became philosophers. Also, some African-Americans learned to become black nationalists in prison, and they became less violent when introduced to Yoga.

Staff Question: Is this an Integral Yoga Institute-sponsored program?

Sri Gurudev: We are going to most of the drug rehabilitation centers and prisons in New Jersey, in New York and in Connecticut. Next month, on the West Coast, in California, I will be visiting two prisons, one in San Francisco and another one somewhere near Santa Cruz.

We Are All Prisoners

Dear friends, it's really a pleasure and a privilege to be here and to serve you by giving you some useful thoughts to benefit your life. And I am very grateful to all the officials here who were so friendly and were so very interested in your welfare. My special thanks should go to my student and your friend, Margabhandu. How do you call him, Marga? I really thank him for bringing me here to meet you all. I heard a lot about you from him, and every time he talks about you his face lights up. He is so happy with your understanding and your interest in growing in a better way. And I hope that, this evening, my ideas will further help you. I know that you have been practicing Yoga, first doing the physical postures, then doing the breathing practices and then doing meditation, also.

You know, a human being is a kind of beautiful mixture–not just onesided. Is he or she a physical being? An emotional being? An intellectual being? A sensual being? And, according to associations with the outside world, is he or she a social being, a communal being, a national or international being? Over and above all these categories, we have another one: a spiritual being. And in the spirit, we are all one. There is no difference between two individuals, because we all have that same spirit, that beautiful element within us. We differ only in our physical bodies, in our emotions, in our habits and in our likes and dislikes. I know that I am talking here in a place called a "prison," or a "correctional institution." How do you use the name now? Do you say "prison" or "correctional institution?" You say prison.

For a long time, I was a bit hesitant to use the word prison. And later on, it dawned on me that, in a way, we are all prisoners. Don't think that only you people who live in this compound, between these walls, are prisoners. Everybody is a prisoner. Our own prison is this body and our senses. We are imprisoned by them. We are imprisoned by our own habits. We are slaves to our habits. So, in that sense, we all make mistakes. But the beauty of the human life is that whenever we realize that we are doing something wrong, we try to reform ourselves, correct ourselves. We want to grow better. We want to show our true inner light. That's why when a person is really beautiful and really behaving well, he or she is called "refined" person. It is that refinement that we all seek. No one is born a saint. Let us know that.

Everyone has, and has had, his or her weakness. It's like a child. When the child is born, it doesn't walk or run. You can't expect the child to win a trophy in the Olympics. The little child just crawls; and when it tries to walk, it slips down. In fact, it falls down hundreds of times. But through its constant attempts, the child will get up and walk and run. And one day, that child may even win a trophy for running. In the same way, we all make mistakes, we all slip. Nobody should be forever condemned for making certain mistakes. Instead, we should be given an opportunity, a helping hand, so that we can correct our mistakes. When you are walking on a slippery road, even a stick helps you. Somebody lends a hand: "Come and walk."

This is the duty of everybody toward our fellow human beings, and institutions like this one are also like that. They are there to give a helping hand. I'm really delighted and fascinated to see real harmony here, to see how well the officers are talking about people. I don't see them here as bosses who are out to punish you. They seem to be very friendly, thinking of your welfare. Maybe, sometimes, their duty would demand them to be a little stricter. But that doesn't mean they are really there to push you, to stand on your neck and to punish you.

I'm a person who visits many prisons in the US and, actually, not only in this country, but also in many other countries. Somehow, I don't know why, I've been chosen for this purpose. Wherever I go, I visit the local prison, but it's only in a few prisons that I see the kind of beautiful harmony, the real understanding that I see here. That's why, when we were walking into the building, I was even telling people that you inmates are really fortunate. I told the reporter, "They must have done good *karma*. That's why they are in this prison instead of in some other prison."

Prison as an *Ashram*

So, let us think that the prison is not a place to punish you; rather, it's a place to reform you, to help you with your own reformation. It's like a hospital. Sometimes, I even go one step further and say that this institution is kind of what we call an *ashram*, a place where you go to do austerities in order to reform. In the same way, you come here to this correctional institution to reform yourself and everyone here is really here to help you. Physically, you get reformed. Mentally, you get reformed. And, then, you go out a totally different person. Why? Because we all want to be reformed; we all want to be good. In fact, that is the purpose of all the different philosophies. Whether a person is religious or not, his or her interest is to be good.

We all want to be praised. We all want that everyone should say: "He's a wonderful man." "She's a wonderful woman." That is the inner urge. Consciously or unconsciously, we all want to be good. But, momentarily, we develop certain weaknesses. We make mistakes. And what is it that, more or less, forces us to make mistakes? It's mainly the mind and its desires. If we could regulate our desires, if we could control our senses a little, then we could avoid many of these mistakes.

Take crimes. The basic reason for all crimes is simply human weakness. It's just at a weak moment that someone commits a crime. Later on, you might regret what you did, realizing, "I shouldn't have done that." That is the true person. But, temporarily, you slip. Why? It's the weakness of the mind. So how can we strengthen ourselves? The entire Yoga system works to make you strong physically and mentally. And why is the physical aspect important? Because even a strong mind cannot express itself in a weak body. It's something like a car that has a nice, well-built engine, a powerful, 440-horse-power engine. But if the wheels are weak, if the brakes are weak, or if the chassis is weak, you can't drive that car fast. The minute you go sixty or seventy miles per hour, the entire body of the vehicle will go to pieces. Another example is a chariot. The horse may run fast, but if the wheels are not in good shape the whole chariot will break down.

Analogously, our body is the chassis, our mind is the engine and it is our heart that pulls the chariot. As the soul, we are the owners of this chariot; we are living in this vehicle. If our journey is to be beautiful and safe, then we must have a good heart, a well-tuned engine, a well-greased and well-fitted body, and a beautiful spirit. Our intelligence is the steam. We control our mind with our intelligence.

Yoga helps us build that strength, that capacity in our mind and body. Many of you might know the expression: a sound mind and a sound body go together (and vice versa). You can easily understand this concept through a simple example. All of sudden, you are frightened of something; the mind becomes fearful. The whole body perspires. You shake. However, the fear is not in the body. It is the mind that experiences the fear. It's a mental action. So why should the body shake? Because the body and mind are so interconnected that you can't separate them. Every gland is a vehicle of the mind. Think of a nice candy. The next minute, your mouth will start salivating. You only thought of the candy. Yet, your salivary glands acted immediately. That shows the connection between the thinking mind and the expressing body. Thus, if you treat one, indirectly you have treated the other.

Yoga Helps us Develop a Sound Body and a Sound Mind

With respect to the body/mind connection, Yoga has a special capacity in treating both the body and mind simultaneously. And that is the reason why all your gymnastic exercises might not have helped you mentally as much as Yoga has helped. That is, even when you do the *Hatha Yoga* poses, you have to bring the mind into a particular situation that claims you. All your excitement and all your restlessness go away. And this is the reason why Yoga is divided into different sections.

First, we focus on the physical body through the Yoga *asanas*, the yogic postures. They're a very, very good way to relax your body by eliminating the toxins. Let us remember that. The body gets tense because of some of the toxins that we put into it through our wrong habits, perhaps by our eating habits or by our smoking habits. Many of the toxins accumulate in the body and that's the cause of tension, rheumatism, arthritis and things like that. That's why all those toxins should be eliminated. We can compare it to wrought iron. Why? Because wrought iron contains a lot of carbon particles. When you burn it, you take the carbon away. It becomes good steel and it bends. It is strong as well as supple. The body is also like that. If the body is filled with toxins, that is, with the waste matter that should have been eliminated, you become rigid, tense. This condition is mainly due to our eating the wrong food, to our eating habits. We don't digest all that we eat. So, take care of that. Eat the right food and the right quantity. Digest it well. When you are hungry, eat. When you are not hungry, do not eat. Then already accumulated toxins are easily eliminated by the *Hatha Yoga* postures, because the postures put gentle pressure on different areas. When you release the toxins, fresh circulation comes into those areas. Blood rushes to those parts. And then the toxins get disturbed, and the circulation carries them away, throwing them out through the pores of the skin or through other organs that excrete toxins. So, through these various *Hatha Yoga* postures (we don't even call them exercise) the elimination process is made very easy.

Just by sitting in different postures or putting the body into different postures, you can apply gentle pressure onto the part that's affected by toxins. Say, for example, your pancreas is not functioning well so you can't digest sugar; you call yourself diabetic. You can do the bow pose–you know, holding the legs behind the body, grabbing onto the legs or feet and a little rocking. The bow pose is a beautiful posture that will give a gentle massage to the pancreas and to the entire abdominal viscera. It tones the pancreas. Once the pancreas is toned, you get your insulin. You don't need to keep on injecting anything to digest your sugar. So whatever sugar you eat gets digested by your own insulin and you become the doctor for your body.

Also, do a little *sarvangasana*, the shoulder stand, which tones your thyroid. Remember, the thyroid gland is, more or less, like the president or the premier of the body. The thyroid controls the entire functioning of the body. If anything goes wrong with the thyroid gland, even the slightest malfunction, it will upset your entire character. All of a sudden, an intelligent person can quickly become erratic. That thyroid can be toned by doing our shoulder stand. In general, these postures help to tone your inner system.

And next is the breathing. By the breathing practices, you build up your lung capacity. You should all know the importance of oxygen to the body. Wherever there is life, you see oxygen. Without oxygen no life exists anywhere. So if we are living beings, we are living because of the oxygen that we breathe in. Every cell needs oxygen. Don't think that only the lungs take oxygen. When you take the breath in, the lungs accept the oxygen. But along with the air and the oxygen that we breathe in, there is another important element that is seldom talked of; in fact, science may not know that much about it. We call it *prana*.

Prana is the vital energy. Air goes into the lungs, bringing oxygen into the lungs. Then, the oxygen gets exchanged with the carbon particles in the veins; it takes carbon and, in return, it gives oxygen and then comes out as carbon dioxide. These carbon particles–that are deposited all over the body and which end up as waste water–are burned by the oxygen and brought to the surface and thrown off. So, the breathing is a very important practice. But the vitality–what we call the vital air–of the *prana*, which is a kind of magnetism or electricity, goes all through the entire body. It charges every cell of your body. In general terms, we say that your cells are being oxygenated. So if you breathe enough and charge your body with more oxygen, your entire body becomes lively. You don't feel a bit of sluggishness anywhere.

In the yogic way of breathing, you take in seven times more air than you take in during your normal breathing, and that means that you're also taking in more oxygen, more vitality. In fact, it has been measured. It's not just a vague theory. In the lab, it has been tested and shown that in your normal breathing, you take in only about 500 cubic centimeters of air and you breathe out the same amount as carbon dioxide. But in the real yogic breathing, you take in 3,700 cubic centimeters of air. This means that you're taking in more than seven times more air. Thus, in every breath you take in seven times more oxygen, more vitality and your cells get revitalized. And that's why you feel all strong and all healthy.

Bring in the Good, the Bad Runs Away

Normally, we try to cure a person by removing the symptoms of a disease. However, in the yogic way, instead of removing the disease, you put in health. That's right; you put in health and the disease goes away. To make an analogy, take a dark room. If you want to make a dark room light, you don't take two sticks and beat the darkness to make it go out. Suppose I put some sticks in your hands and say, "Come on, beat the darkness away. Let there be light." You will probably end up beating each other, because, in the darkness, you don't see anything. Instead, you can bring in just one candle and the whole room is lit immediately. That's what. Bring in the good and the bad runs away. It's only a matter of substitution. We can't always beat the bad and drive it away. What we can do is to replace the bad with the good. In fact, that's why we see the benefits manifesting here. Because *maya* [the illusion of the reality of sensory experience] brought in the good, therefore the bad is automatically going away without even saying goodbye to you. Everybody is happy without even your effort.

Yes, do the right thing and the wrong goes.

The reality is that one wrong cannot be corrected by another wrong. Take heroin addiction, for example. When I go to drug rehabilitation centers, I talk to people about heroin addiction. Heroin addiction is wrong. And what are doctors doing to remove this wrong? They're giving methadone. They're putting in another wrong. In other words, instead of putting in one poison, the heroin addicts are putting in another poison. Then, they get addicted to that poison. Instead, we say, remove the poison by putting in some nectar. The most wonderful way to charge your system with nectar is just to breathe. Breath is our life. You are charging the entire body with life. And again, remember that breath not only builds up the body, but it also builds up the mind. If you regulate the breath, you have regulated the mind.

To give an example: suppose somebody looks at you and calls you a bad word or says, "You are a dirty fool," or something like that. He or she is only using a word, isn't that so? It's only a sound, right? There's nothing there but a sound. However, that sound gives you a meaning, and you get really disturbed. You become angry. Immediately, you get heated up and your whole body burns. Your blood boils. Just a little agitation of the mind and the whole body comes agitated. And what happens to your breath? That's the point I want to make. Will you be breathing slowly, calmly when you are angry? The other person is only using a word, but why are you breathing so heavily, as though you've been outside moving tons of things, working hard for eight hours? The secret is that agitation of the mind brings agitation of the breath. So we take the clue, saying, "Okay; so to calm the mind, calm the breath." And vice versa.

You take the clue from there. When the mind is agitated, the breath is agitated. When the breath is calmed, the mind is calmed. Am I right? That is why when you do the slow, simple deep breathing, your mind is so peaceful. We even use this breathing practice before meditation. Sometimes you do alternate nostril breathing for awhile and, then, you don't even need to alternate. Just sit quietly. Breathe slowly, in and out. Let the mind be attentive to the breath. However restless you are, in two or three minutes, you will feel like a baby. You are so calm. That's why breath is an important point. As a matter of fact, in Yoga, breathing takes care of many things. It burns out all the impurities of the body. It calms the mind. When the mind is calm, the advantage is that you become strong. Imagine that you keep on working without any sleeping. Very soon, you will die. Am I right? You know why? Because there's no rest.

Continuous work means exhausting one's energy. There's no time to rebuild. That's why nature has provided us with sleep. When we sleep, we are relaxed. Every cell is rebuilt.

To give another example, there is one organ in our body that works constantly. What is that organ? The heart. The heart is the one organ that functions constantly from birth to death. If the heart stops, the person is dead. Yet, with all the constant functioning, do you think that the heart takes rest? Does it take ever rest? No. When you sleep, the heart still functions. But I say that it takes rest. When? You know, normally, doctors describe the heartbeat as: "Lub dub, lub dub." Is it not so? The valves work as, "Lub dub, lub dub . . ." However, if you really, carefully notice the rhythm of the heartbeat or actually ask the doctors, the doctors will say, "Lub dub *pause*, lub dub *pause*, lub dub *pause*." The pause indicates total rest for the heart. But in between every lub and dub, there is a momentary pause. The heart is rebuilt within that pause. It takes a rest between every lub and dub.

Why is the rest necessary? When we rest enough, we gather energy. We rebuild. That is why we allow the mind to rest in meditation; we're not working the mind. We calm the mind with the breath and then, just let go, let it be. Simply let it be there and observe what's happening. The mind rests in meditation. Even a minute of good rest is enough for the mind to become strong.

So to repeat: by the Yoga postures and by relaxing, you eliminate the toxins from the body and you bring rest to the body. By breathing, you calm the mind. And by meditation, you give rest to the mind. When the mind and body rest like that, they regain strength. They get rejuvenated. That's why, after a few minutes of relaxation, however tired you may be, you will notice how relaxed and healthy you are when you get up, as though you have gotten eight hours of sleep. That is because of the perfect rest. If you know this trick and apply this rest in between your activities, you can retain your physical and mental strength. And when you are really that strong, you become the master of your mind and you become the master of your senses.

Only a weak person makes mistakes, as I told you in the beginning. If you are strong mentally, you don't need to make mistakes. It's a weak mind that gets you into trouble. Say for instance, you get upset when somebody annoys you. If you are weak-minded, immediately you give the person a nice, big hit. The next minute you cry, "What did I do?" But it's too late. Now you have to run and hide. How many crimes are committed by this type of momentary weakness? If only we could get over that momentary weakness and just smile at the other person's mistakes: "Poor guy. He didn't know what he was doing; let it go." If you learn just to forgive the person, you don't get angry and you don't commit a crime. So, it's just a mental weakness and most crimes are committed that way.

On the other hand, you may say that some crimes are well planned and plotted. But even that is a kind of weakness. Based on a weakness, you plan to commit a crime. That's a weakness in a different direction. The purpose of Yoga is to help us become the masters of our own bodies and minds by making our bodies and minds healthy, pure and clean.

The Good Life = The Selfless Life

In addition to the Yoga practices we also recommend a good day-to-day life. What do we mean by that? We mean a life free from selfishness. All our troubles–not only on the individual level, but also on the national and political levels–are caused by peoples' selfishness. People want everything for themselves. They don't think of the other person. In fact, if you put the other person first and yourself next, you would never commit a crime. All our lies, all our thefts, all our crimes are committed because of our selfishness. If you could learn to be selfless and dedicated, then there would be no room to get disturbed, to get disappointed and to commit any crime.

Furthermore, if anybody complains of being disappointed, I say, "You are the cause of your disappointment. Don't blame anybody. Why? Because you made an *appointment* and that appointment got *dissed*, isn't that so?

What is disappointment? Disappointment is an appointment that got disturbed. That is disappointment, correct? *Disappointment.*

Without an appointment can it ever get dissed? If there is no appointment, then there can never be a dis-appointment. Do you understand my point? So, who or what is the cause of our disappointments? Our own appointments. When you say, "I'm disappointed," it means that you have made an appointment: "Such and such a thing will happen to me." Then, if it doesn't happen, you say, "I am disappointed."

Thus, the cause of the disappointment is the appointment. "I wanted something. I didn't get it. So, I am disappointed." When you feel disappointed, you look for a cause: "Who is the cause of my disappointment?" You don't blame yourself. But if you really analyzed it, you would realize that it's you who is to be blamed for having made that appointment. Unfortunately, though, we don't face up to our own mistakes. We immediately blame somebody else: "That fellow is the cause of my disappointment." And the next thing is that you're angry. You hate him. Then, you're apt to do some harm to him. That's why everyone should learn to lead a dedicated life, a selfless life.

Always think of others. Serve others. Help others. When you live for others, you will get help. In fact, you will get everything. Take, for example, an apple tree. An apple tree gives a lot of fruit. It just offers fruit to others. And because the tree offers so much fruit, you take good care of it. Likewise, if you are a useful citizen, the people around you take good care of you. "Oh, she is very useful. We get a lot of help from her. She must be kept in good shape." Everyone will take good care of you. You don't even need to worry about your own needs. That is the advantage of leading a dedicated life. That will eliminate all the crime. Don't think that only the people who are caught and who are in a prison like this one are the criminals. There are political criminals, and even to wage war against other countries is a crime. Why? "My country should prosper, only my country." That kind of thinking reflects a kind of national selfishness. Why not the other country also? Instead, if every country would think of the benefit of the other countries, it wouldn't even matter if we didn't have enough food to eat, we would ship all our food to them because we would want them to eat well. Until we learn to think and to act that way, there will always be wars and crime.

But where to begin? You may all ask, "Why doesn't that person do that? Why doesn't this individual do that? The congressman should do that. The senators should do that. The president should do that." My question is: Why not you? You begin first. At least, in your life, you will find everything beautiful. Your life will be balanced and happy. You will never get disappointed. You will learn to lead a beautiful life. In fact, it is to learn that we are here. Don't think this is a place of punishment. I really don't like to think that a prison is a place for punishment. Neither the people who live here nor the authorities who serve here should think in that way. You are not being punished. You are being given opportunities to reform yourselves, to think of your mistakes and to undo what you have done.

No, you're not being punished. Remember, many great people, sages and saints, became sages and saints because of their prison life. If you look at history, you will see that many individuals came out of prison as great people. Am I right? That's what. So don't think that prison is a dirty place or a place of punishment, no. We are being reformed, being given opportunities to reform. This place is here just to help you. But if you don't cooperate and if you don't want to reform yourself, then it becomes a difficult place.

So, the only thing is to understand why you are here: how can I make use of this place? Then you make the best use of it. And you come out as a well-reformed, beautiful, useful citizen.

Yoga makes you think of all these things. Yoga is not just a few sets of Yoga postures or even breathing practices. It's a way of life. It enables you to be good and it enables you to do good and to be totally relaxed, happy and healthy always, to lead a life without any disappointments, without any anxiety. I have seen many, many people who were in prison and who learned this yogic way of life and came out as beautiful people. In my forty years or so of service, I have seen many prisoners, in many different countries. In fact, I am still in communication with many of them. Some of them are good farmers. Some of them are good ministers. They are reformers. That's why I would like to say: please take this opportunity; use it for your benefit; and don't even think that you are being punished here.

The Cause and Effect Principle

Actually, some of you may be here without even having committed a crime. In this regard, there is another important point that I would like to make. Many people say, "I haven't done anything. Why am I here?" Certainly, your own conscience would tell you. If you really know that you have not done anything and, yet, you are here, I would like to remind you of one thing: there is always a cause for an effect. Cause and effect are inseparable. It's something like, all of a sudden, I get a cramp, an acute pain in the stomach. You ask, "What is it?" And I reply, "I don't know. I haven't done anything wrong. I didn't eat anything bad all day or even yesterday." However, you may have eaten something bad the week before, and it took this much time for it to come out and to create some trouble.

Cancer, for example, is not produced overnight by one cigarette. It takes tons of cigarettes to produce cancer, not merely one extra-long, 100-millimeter cigarette. It takes millions of millimeters; it takes time. So, if you wonder how you got cancer, you have to think, "I did something in the past. I am facing the effect now." In the same way, if you are experiencing some kind of suffering now and, yet, you are innocent, you would have done something before, maybe years before. Or, as we believe, you might have even done something in a past life. You probably escaped because you had enough money or you had good lawyers who argued well. In any case, no matter what the reason might have been, you got out of it.

But God's law waits. You can't escape from God's law, although you might escape from human law. God says, "Okay, wait. I'll give you a reward at the proper time." Then, all of a sudden one day, for nothing, you will get caught. If you understand this process, you won't even blame the witness or you won't have any grudge against the witness who gave the evidence that put you into prison. The witness was only an instrument used for you to undergo the suffering for something that you did long before. That is what we call the *karma* theory. Whatever you do you have to face one day or other.

Therefore, suffering will never come to you if you are innocent, if you have not done anything, for cosmic law, is more understanding and more powerful than human law. Human law might make mistakes. But divine law, cosmic law never makes mistakes. If you accept it that way: "Well, probably I haven't done anything now, but I might have done something before. Anyway, my fate, my destiny, my *karma* brought me here. Let me get clean," then you will be peaceful here and you will make the best use of the condition that you find yourself in. Otherwise, you might be carrying a grudge.

Sometimes, you are annoyed with the officers here. Or sometimes you feel, "That fellow! It is that witness, that key witness who put me here. Wait, just let me get out!" How many people think that way? As soon as they walk out of prison, they commit another crime. They say, "It doesn't matter. Even if I end up going back to prison, I'm going to dispose of him or her." But what have you gained? You haven't gained anything. If the witness has really committed some mistake, God will take care of it. His or her own *karma* will take care of it. You don't need to worry about it. We are not here to punish everybody. It's not possible for us to punish everybody. That is a common law. So don't carry a grudge against anybody. Accept what has come and purge it out.

To make another analogy, you walk on the road; you stumble on a small stone and fall down. Do you get up, go back and hit the stone because you stumbled? Think like that. That witness was a stone on the way. You stumbled on him or her and you fell down. In truth, there's no room for us to harbor any hatred toward anybody. Of course, it's easy to love our friends and it's hard to love our enemies. But if we understand it in this light, then there's nobody who is an enemy in our world. We can be friends to everybody.

Well, I could keep on talking to you. I see your faces, and you are really deeply receiving these teachings. But I don't want to overburden you, so I will give you enough time to digest what you've heard. Maybe if your sheriff and our officers permit it and if there is still a little time, you can probably ask me a few questions if you like. I'll try to answer you.

To Sleep, Perchance to Dream

Question: Why do we dream?

Sri Gurudev: We dream because of our anxieties. There are many unfulfilled desires in our daily life. We don't lead a contented life. "I want this and that and that and that." All those unfulfilled desires slowly slip into the subconscious mind. We may forget them consciously, but they are there waiting in the subconscious. Once you sleep, the subconscious mind comes to the surface. And that is what you call the astral body. Then, the subconscious mind gets satisfaction by going around in the dream world and satisfying itself of all that it wanted and what you couldn't do consciously. See?

Suppose you just wanted to go eat an apple from someone's garden. Consciously, you couldn't do it, because it's barred. The garden is fenced and it's an offense. So, when you sleep, your subconscious mind will go and eat all the apples from that garden. To understand this point more clearly, you can imagine a steam boiler. A steam boiler has an exhaust, a safety valve for when the given pressure goes up too high. In a way, the subconscious mind takes the safety valve of your dream and goes out and experiences everything.

If such desires are not fulfilled in the dream state, you will really go mad. Furthermore, if you, in your conscious life, don't put all those desires and anxieties into the subconscious mind, the subconscious mind won't become fearful and then you don't dream that much. But if we take care of our daily life, then sleep comes easily; we can sleep like a baby. That's why I say that merely doing practices is not enough. You have to take care of every minute of your life. In fact, you have to take care of every thought, because the human being is a thinking being. *As you think, so you become.* So, if you can regulate your thoughts, you become a wonderful person. Otherwise, your own thoughts bring you all kinds of trouble and suffering.

Karma Yoga

Question: Can you tell us the seven steps of karma?
Sri Gurudev: Well, there are no seven steps as such. No. There are no particular different steps as such of *karma*. Every action has its own reaction. When you face the reaction, you call it a *karma*. Certain *karmas* bring the reaction immediately. For example, if I put my finger into the fire, I get the reaction immediately. I don't need to wait for the next day. But if I put something wrong into the stomach, maybe after three days it will burn there. That is the difference between the *karmas*. Some are instantaneous. Some wait. There aren't any fast and fixed rules about *karma*. We don't always know what the consequence of a particular action will be or when it will express itself. Only the Cosmic Consciousness knows. And all we can do is to take care of *karma*, take care of what we do. If we sow the right things, we reap the right things.

Life After Death

Question: We were living before and we will live after also. The soul is eternal. So, what is death? Does it refer only to the physical body? Suppose a friend dies back in your hometown. People say, "He's dead and gone." What does that mean, "He's dead and gone?" Where is he? He is dead and gone where?
Sri Gurudev: What is dead and what is gone? The dead matter is still in the box there. That's where she is buried. And where did she go? She's gone. It's the physical body dying. But all your desires, all your aspirations are in a different body, which you call the astral body. That body doesn't die that easily. That body goes on taking different bodies until it exhausts all it desires.

In the Western religions, they sometimes say that this is the only birth and there is no reincarnation or anything like that. But, because questions arise, I may have to touch on that point. The only answer I could give is that if this is the only birth and we never lived before and we are not going to live after, then the soul is not immortal. Another proof is that if we are all just coming for the first time into this world, why should we have all these differences? We are all born from the same factory, produced by the same factory. Why then should one be born with all one's bodily functions in good shape while others are born with different handicaps? Some people are born blind, some are born deaf. Why all these deformities, then? What is the cause for that? Even twins seem to have two different kinds of characters. What is the cause? They come out of the same mother and have the same father. Why should they have different temperaments? The answer is that they bring to this life something of their past lives, and they will continue. This process gives us an opportunity to correct ourselves and to decide what we can be later on. If we do the right thing, we will enjoy the right birth later on.

I have experienced many aspects of life. I have been a student, a householder and I've worked in many business fields. But somehow, in many of those areas, I experienced a lot of disappointment and anxiety. Like most of you, I tried to blame others: "He was the cause. She was the cause." Then, later on, I realized, "What is this? I can't always be putting the blame on others' shoulders. If I had acted another way, I would not have to face this situation." So I learned to analyze myself and my motivations. I tried to find out whether I was the cause, in any way, of my actions, my anxieties, my greed, my disappointment. I realized that all my suffering was due to my own selfishness. I wanted everything to happen for me and whenever anybody got in my way, I hated him, I got disappointed by her. The more that I acquired, the more greedy I got. I wanted more and more. There were no limitations. Then I asked myself, "What is this life that I'm leading? What am I going to be satisfied with? The more I get, the more I want. There's no end. So, okay, no more! Let me be content with what I have. And even with that, let me use it for others. Whatever it is, whether it be money or other possessions or my intelligence or my physical energy, I'll just use it.

Even our coming here itself is an example. For how many years, for how many months have you been coming, Marg? Yes. That's how I train people. "Come on, go! Do! This is your service to your own fellow human beings, your brothers and your sisters. Go do it. Don't demand any money. Don't sell anything. Don't make it a business. You do it. If they really see something beautiful, and if they feel that you should be rewarded or that you should be given something for your effort, let them give it." Certainly the world has a soft corner for everything. People recognize good things. Even the mind and heart of the worst person has a nice part. If you just use a nice word and love that person, he or she will realize it. An animal understands your love. Can't a human being? So, I came to feel that by love, by loving service you can conquer the whole world. You can be a good friend to all. You can be always happy. And I'm enjoying that for the past so many years. I'm never disappointed.

Also, because of my peace of mind, I don't even fall physically sick. I am always healthy and happy. I seldom go to a doctor. I don't even remember when I went to a doctor in the past thirty or forty years. What else do you want in this life? Just be peaceful. Enjoy the world. Serve it. Every given minute be happy. That's *divine life*. That's what we all should enjoy. That's our birthright.

When we don't understand that and when we misuse our life and capacities and energies, then we pay a price for it. In many ways, we violate nature's law. Take the case of breathing, which I spoke about earlier. The oxygen that you breathe in gives you life. Correct? So if you want to live a healthy life, you have to breathe in oxygen. Do you pay for your oxygen? It's all free, is it not? Nature gives it to you. Or you can say that God gives it to you. But you don't want that free gift, that oxygen. You want to pay for your poison: "Come on, give me an extra-long millimeter cigarette." And you inhale all the nicotine. Yet, you want to purify your lungs and be healthy. The fact is: Nectar is free. You reject it. Poison is expensive. You buy it. Naturally, we have to pay the price for it. Nature, itself, punishes us: "Hey, I am giving you nectar. You reject it, and you are going after poison with your hardearned money. Certainly, you have to suffer. What can I do? You did it and you deserve it." You see, you can't blame anybody else for that. I'm just giving you an example.

Likewise, in our life, we make many mistakes. We violate nature's law. Observe nature, everywhere. A flower doesn't expect anything from you in return. It smiles at you, gives you all nice things. It doesn't even ask you for a thank you. It's just there. What a lovely thing to see and to learn from. But in our case, even if we do one little nice thing, we expect thanks. And if she doesn't thank me: "What a dirty person! She doesn't even know how to say thank you. How ungrateful!" If the entire nature were to say that to us, then we would be 100 percent ungrateful. Then the food would curse us. The air would curse us. Look how we pollute the air. Still, we get some fresh air from some corner and the air doesn't curse us. The entire nature lives selflessly. We should learn from the very nature. Nature, itself, is a book. We should study and learn from the plants, from the trees, from the fruit, from the sun, from the rain. Rain pours out to everybody, whether one is a rich person or a poor person. It doesn't make any difference. We should learn to be like that. In fact, we should not even discriminate between friend and foe–this person is our neighbor and that person is some other fellow; this person is our countryman and that person is from some other country.

Be Selfless

What's more, because of discrimination, our attitude is: "My countrymen must enjoy life, so I have to get everything I can from other countries; and maybe that means that I'll have to drop bombs on a neighboring country or on some another country." But if you love your neighbor as yourself, then why can't you love the neighboring country as your country? It all has to do with human greed; it's the selfishness of the human beings that is the cause of all this trouble. That's why, speaking on the religious level, every religion pinpoints this teaching: Be selfless. Be dedicated. If you look at the Cross, what is the symbolic message that you get? Sacrifice. Every religious person, every seeker, every prophet, every sage has sacrificed him- and herself for humanity. That's why you respect and you worship them, you adore them, you want to follow them. A selfish person is never followed or respected. Well, maybe as long as he's in power, you salute him, probably out of fear, not out of gratitude. But a selfless person is respected by the whole world. Wherever she goes she's respected. That's what we should learn.

Try for even one week to be like this–a sample week, a selfless week. For the whole week, feel, "Let me be selfless. Let me always give, give, give and love, love, love." If you really don't get any benefit, don't enjoy that week, okay, go back to your old pattern, your old behavior. I don't know whether in this country you have a kind of courtesy week. In our country, all of a sudden, the police will come up and say, "It is courtesy week for the police. We'll be extra nice to you." They won't say, "Hey, stop." No, they'll say, "Please stop." It's called courtesy week. In India and in Ceylon [Sri Lanka] we had that. All the officers would be very courteous for one week and everybody enjoyed it.

I see courtesy here in this facility and I see beauty here. As I mentioned before, you should have heard how your officers were talking about you. I don't know whether I am revealing any secrets, but they were all praising you: "They are wonderful people. They are changing." I am also a little jealous. They are praising Marg. I am proud of him and you all. You are really bringing glory to the great science of Yoga.

You don't know really what you are doing. But I do know that. I was really moved with emotion when I heard Marg say, "Yoga is helping them so much." It's only a beginning. Now I am looking forward to serving more people through his breakthrough. He's really breaking through. Very soon, we will make the whole country filled with yogis. I think America is the place for it.

Thank you all for this beautiful evening. God bless you and peace be with you. *OM Shanti. OM Tat Sat.*

Danbury Prison
Danbury, Connecticut, March 26, 1972

In the summer of 1969, Kanniah Cohen and a couple of other disciples set up an Integral Yoga Institute in Hartford, Connecticut. It wasn't too long before Kanniah started offering Integral Yoga classes at Danbury Prison in Danbury, Connecticut. The response was wonderful and, as in other prisons where Integral Yoga was being taught, student-inmates invited Gurudev to come to speak with them. On March 26, 1972, Gurudev spoke at Danbury to an audience of more than a hundred inmates. In this correctional facility, as in every other one in which he spoke, Gurudev made sure to call attention to what is probably the most essential–and, perhaps, the most controversial–aspect of the prison experience, and that is: reformation.

The Prison Repair Shop

Friends, I am really very delighted to be here, to meet you and to share some of my thoughts. I have heard a lot about you and about your interest in this Yoga philosophy through my dear son and student, Sri Kanniah. I am sure that he has stimulated your keen interest and that is the reason why you are all here this evening to see me.

First of all, I am thankful to Sri Kanniah for having brought me to you and for having created this interest and for having set a good example. I know that, normally, you begin your classes with a little *OM* and a little chanting. So, shall we have a couple of minutes to do the *OM Shanthi* chant? I request that you all follow me. And I request that you repeat the chant, because the repetition of that very beautiful word *Shanthi* brings peace. The word creates a feeling. Keep on repeating *Shanthi, Shanthi* and you will feel peace.

Now, I'm fully aware that I am sitting here in a place where people come to correct themselves, to reform themselves, because they needed it. The experience could be probably compared to a repair shop, where something is brought to put it into the proper shape. In fact, when we talk about correcting something or somebody, we call it "reforming." We are supposed to be in a particular shape but, somehow, we failed to be in this form. Something went wrong, so we are putting ourselves back into the original shape. That is why we even use the words "reform" and "reforming." Understand, it is not that the reformer is going to do something new to you; rather, he is just putting you back into your original state. You were well-formed and, somehow, you got de-formed, and so you have to be re-formed. And that is what we expect to happen in places like this.

Don't think that this type of institution is the only reformatory or correctional place. This is a place created especially for that purpose by men. But in fact, the entire world, the very nature is a correctional institution. Don't think that in the outside world you are free to do anything you want. How many people commit mistakes and yet don't find themselves in such institutions as this one? In these cases, their own conscience corrects them: they are not happy.

So, who should be happy? The one who is in the proper shape. To make an analogy, when you fall sick, except in some exceptional cases, you are not sent to a doctor by force. There is no need for such force to bring back your ease. And what is the meaning of disease–*dis-ease*? A disturbed ease. That is what is called disease, and what the doctor does is to put you back in that ease which you somehow disturbed. Here, though, in this correctional institution, the correction is a moral correction. When you go into a place of worship, that place is also a correctional institution. You have fallen from your true nature. You have forgotten that you are the child of God. You have fallen from that understanding. All through life, we slip from our original state and are, again and again, reformed and placed back into our original state. If we could think in these terms, then I don't think anyone would complain about being in an institution like this. We are simply being corrected.

It is not that this institution is a place where you are punished for your mistakes. I don't like the word "punishment." When you eat something wrong and you get a stomachache, God doesn't punish you. You may undergo some suffering. But the intention is not punishment; the intention is to help you. Why not treat this place as a monastery, a place where you are being helped, where you will come out as a beautiful person, a beautiful citizen, pure in heart, loved by God.

Of course, God is always blessing us. We don't need to ask God to bless us. But we must be able to receive those blessings. So, who is loved by God? God loves the one who is pure in heart; the one who is clean. To make another analogy, only a radio in proper shape will receive the music being aired. Does that mean that the music is not in all the boxes? In the same way, we are all receivers. And when we keep ourselves in proper shape, we receive the blessings. God never dislikes or punishes or hurts anybody.

Speaking about God

Speaking about God, there is even doubt about who that
God is. Is God in heaven somewhere? According to the yogic
thinking, God is formless and nameless. God is omnipresent. But
without a form and a name, we cannot understand God. So, for
the sake of limited individuals, God appears as a limited person.
As we expand our understanding, our understanding of God also
expands. When you become infinite, you realize the infinite God.
And what limits you? Your own thinking limits you. You identify
yourself with limited thinking, not with spirit. You talk in terms of
the body or in terms of your mental capacity. You talk in terms of
your occupations. You combine yourself with what you do or with
the ideas that you gather in your brain. With these combinations,
you limit yourself. But the true you is above these things. The body
and mind are your instruments. You are the spirit, which you call
the life or the soul. And it is this spirit that is the image of God.
Realization of the true Self is the real self only. When we forget
that and when we identify ourselves with all these things, then we
have slipped down from our original state. That is the beginning of
all our troubles.

Then how to realize the Kingdom of Heaven? The Kingdom of
Heaven is here. To realize it, you need the help of the mind. The
mind is like a mirror. It can reflect your true nature. Making the
mind calm and serene is the purpose of all religions. As long as we
are impure, we lose the capacity to see God in us and outside of us,
too. But why should the mind lose its purity? By nature it should
be pure. When God created the human being, God created the
mind and the body, too. Then why should the body fall sick? By our
wrong food, by excess usage of the body, by using the vital energy
from the body or, sometimes, by not doing anything (daily activity
is necessary). Without these basic requirements, the body might
fall sick.

The main issue, though, is eating the wrong food, food that
leaves toxins in the body. Also, if our thoughts are not clean, they
will disturb the mind. A disturbed mind is a sick mind. In fact,
anything that comes into you is your food. There is a famous

Chinese saying: "See no evil; hear no evil; speak no evil." And this proverb is symbolized in the figures of three monkeys shown with their eyes, ears and mouths closed. These monkeys teach the other monkeys–probably only a monkey will listen to a monkey. It's important to remember, in other words, that everything that you experience in your life is your food.

Now you're probably thinking, "What should I do? I see hundreds of things around me, but I don't see anything good. I wake up to the music of a garbage truck. When I walk on the street, I'm not really walking; I'm rocking and rolling because of the music that I listen to." Actually, I don't condemn that. Should I say that rock and roll music is bad? Nothing is bad. Then how can I say, "See no evil, Hear no evil, Speak no evil"? It seems to be contradictory. But the evil doesn't exist outside. It is the mind that is evil. Just this morning, I was turning the pages of a book, *Shintoism*, I think. I read that when you walk in front of someone and see a thief in him, know that you see a thief in you. Everybody is a mirror. An evil mind will always see evil things.

The *Bhagavad Gita* says that it is your own mind that is your enemy or your friend. In other words, you project the entire world outside. What is that evil then? What is that basic thing that disturbs the mind? Analyze it: "Why am I disturbed?" Question it. You will say: "It's because of him or her." Easy. You try to put the blame on somebody. He is the cause, or she is the cause. But that is not the right answer. All of a sudden, that person disturbed you? Did *you* do anything? If you really analyze the situation, you will, ultimately, come to this one truth: you wanted something to happen just for you–"I wanted this to happen." In fact, most crimes are committed because of selfishness. You think, "*I* must have him" or "She must be *mine.*" *I and mine.* That comes first. If we could only get rid of that selfishness. What's more, it may not even be individual selfishness; it may be communal: "My community wants this, so I can throw a bomb on the other one." That is national pride. But a person who wants to enjoy peace will always think of the entire world. Yes, think in terms of the world, not in terms of your town, your community. Otherwise, you are making yourself little. If the whole world is yours, then you become infinite. When you think in terms of the infinite, then your mind becomes infinite.

We limit ourselves even in the name of God. People fight even in the name of God. How many countries fight in the name of God? Hindus and Muslims are fighting. And what is happening in Ireland? Two countries following the same prophet and reading the same Bible are killing each other. Is it in the Bible or in the prophet? No, it is in the mind. God created everybody equal. Even dogs and cats are created by God. Why is it that only human beings commit such violence against each other? Because we seem to be intelligent but perverted. Because we don't follow the essential principles taught by our religions.

The basic teaching of all religions is to lead a selfless life, to feel that the entire world is made up of your own brothers and sisters. Dedication is essential. And sacrifice. Sacrificing what? Sacrificing selfishness. Lord Jesus is worshipped because he sacrificed himself on the Cross. What makes him great? It is the sacrifice. So don't do anything for your sake. A selfless, dedicated person will always be happy. As such, he or she will never commit any crimes, never need any correction. It's a real opportunity for us.

Actually, I envy your place. I want an *ashram* like this. What a serene, blissful atmosphere! You are very well protected. They see that you are well taken care of. In my life, anyone can disturb me when I am meditating. It's really a matter of attitude. If you think you are in a prison, then you will be. Remember, if you just change the attitude of mind, you change the prison into a monastery. This can be your heaven if you see it like that.

Take, for example, a shirt. If it is clean, will it go to the laundry? No. But once the shirt goes to the laundry, how will the laundryman clean it? He will soak it in water, rub it and squeeze it. He will put it into all kinds of troubles. He is not angry with the shirt, though. He is angry with the dirt. He is trying to separate the dirt from the material. After he is through, the shirt may have some wrinkles. If so, you have to apply a hot iron. Then it becomes straight and clean and ready to be worn. This institution is an extraspecialized laundry. It may not happen quick as a wink. It depends on how much dirt you have accumulated, how much you allow yourself to be cleaned, to be purged out. If you think along these lines, you will become perfectly clean; but if you don't, you will hate everything. You will want to get out of prison in order to take revenge. Maybe in six months, you will be back here, again. If only you could think in the right way; then, you won't be back.

A student of mine was sent to prison as a result of being framed. Before he was convicted, he spoke to me, asking: "What am I to do?" I replied, "You might have done something before, but you escaped from facing the consequences that time." *Karma.* And don't think that the person who did escape judgment will always be free. The ultimate judgment is there. Whenever you get into some kind of suffering, think that it is occurring because you did something incorrect sometime before and you escaped facing the consequences. To understand this philosophy, we must believe in reincarnation, that is, that the cause of the conditions in this lifetime is linked to actions performed in a previous incarnation.

To explain, some children are born blind and some religious people say it is because of the parents. This would be like putting your finger in the fire and someone else getting burned. The answer is that the condition has to do with something that the children had done before. In other words, before the children faced the reaction of their actions, they lost their bodies. Sometimes people commit all kinds of crimes, and they never get caught or anything; but in the next birth, something will be waiting for them. *What you sow you must reap.* If we can understand and accept that, we will not begrudge suffering; we will accept it; and we will be cleaned of selfishness. But until we get rid of selfishness, we will continue to get robbed and robbed. The key to finding permanent peace is dedication. Nobody can disturb the peace of someone who is dedicated.

Again, as I said before, our true nature is divine, the image of God. However, we have forgotten our true nature, and for us to understand the infinite nature of God, He or She or It must come to us through a finite person. Our wrong identification–that is, not identifying with our divine nature–occurs because of our selfishness. Every selfish act disturbs our mind. Dedication should rule our lives. Of course, this teaching is only for human beings, because the other creatures are already living dedicated lives. Go ask an apple tree, "Why are you here?"

"Sir, I am here to bring forth fruits."

"Don't you even taste a few?"

"No."

The forbidden fruit is not somewhere in the Garden of Eden. Because man wants to taste his own fruits, he gets into trouble. Offer your fruits to others. Would you feed a tree that eats its own fruits? Ask a candle, "Why are you burning?" "To give you light." "But you are dying." "It doesn't matter." There is no prison for anything but human beings. Only we make these mistakes. Furthermore, don't think that money, position, power will make you happy. Those who come to the topmost power may even get assassinated. And the more money you make, the more tax you pay. The richest man is the one who lives for the sake of others. Whatever you do, do it for your own peace or for the peace of others. It is the same.

So, what is this that I hear, that your immediate guru teaches all about postures? I've been telling you about the mind and your immediate guru Sri Kanniah has been telling you about the body. Take care of your body, too. Peace is your goal. Take care of anything that disturbs your peace. We don't say that you should just accept everything. If you really can't accept something, express it in a peaceful way. Everywhere we find violence, even in the universities. How can we get peace by throwing bombs? Don't think of force always. No power is greater than your own. Physically and mentally we should find peace. We should have faith in God.

I think I have said enough.

Question: You said we must accept things as they come. I cannot accept my children getting hungry and getting an inferior education while millions of tons of food are being dumped into the ocean.

Sri Gurudev: How can you reform? You can agitate, but not by violence. When I say accept, I don't mean that you should accept everything. About sending people to war: don't accept it. If you have faith in your philosophy, then you will accept whatever comes. If you really send out good thoughts, others will change. When you don't believe in killing and violence out there, then how can you create violence in here? No country has achieved its real freedom by violence. You may have won a victory, but you have hatred. I can't say that you have won a victory by having external enemies. The real victory comes out of love. And the country that loses today might come back again to obtain a victory. We should have patience. Instead of immediately finding fault with others, a little patient analysis will help us.

Question: How can one begin to attain infinite knowledge of the self and is there more than one way?

Sri Gurudev: There is more than one way, but they are all in the mind. To undo all obstacles, you can give everything to God, saying that "nothing is mine." How can we begin to think this way? You have to change the thinking. On one side, you think of the benefits of changing; on the other side, you think of the harm you do by not changing. You talk in terms of your body. Who becomes young or old? It is the body. You have tied yourself to the body; you must separate yourself from it. When the mind is disturbed, you can separate yourself from the thoughts and know that you are the knower of that condition. It takes time, but if a person wants it, he or she can achieve it. It is the only way to find everlasting peace. Whatever it may be, you have to liberate yourself. Those who follow the *bhakti*, or devotional path say that there is God and that everything belongs to God. Go and give it away. Either you offer it to God or to the community at large. But this will happen only if you are convinced that it is the best way. You can give what you have. And if you find peace, at least that part of the world finds peace. Peace talks fail because there seems to be no peace in the minds of those who talk at the peace talks. Charity begins at home. Everything begins at home, including jealousy and hatred.

Question: Suppose that you don't need to be reformed? Suppose that you are put in here by a frameup?

Sri Gurudev: You might have done something before. If people can frame you, then they are great gods.

Question: If I don't feel like a piece of dirty laundry, then what?

Sri Gurudev: The very reason you are here is because you are dirty. If you were not dirty, you would not be here. You have to think, "Have I done anything wrong to make my mind dirty?" But remember, that is only your conscious mind. What about the subconscious? Without a cause, there is no effect. The reason you are here is that you have had some cause before. The higher consciousness knows why you are here.

Question: Where do I begin to go in a positive direction?

Sri Gurudev: Now you are here. It is a fact. By accepting your situation, you can make use of it and get through it well. Something has happened. Why make it worse? If you agitate, you will make the cell experience more difficult for yourself.

Question: How do I find out what is God's will?

Sri Gurudev: There is a natural law. When you do something, it is nature's law. Either you analyze and say you have done something before, or you say it is God's will. When the human being becomes self-centered, then he or she does something against nature's law, against God's will. God has not created evil. There is nothing such as evil. *You* make it evil. Take electricity. There is an outlet here. Is it good or devilish? If you plug in a lamp, it is good. If you plug in your finger, it is devilish. It is you. By your correct approach, you make the world a heaven or a hell. If you feel it is good to kill someone, you can but, then you must accept other people's will. Human beings are always a mixture of good and bad. Only one part is bad. In the same way, a rose is good, a thorn is bad. Perhaps, you may have used your thorn.

Question: Isn't Yoga a form of self-hypnosis?

Sri Gurudev: Yoga is more a form of selfcorrection. You can call it self-hypnosis. Humans are thinking beings. They live as they think. Some doctors wanted to prove the effect of body and mind over life. They took a prisoner condemned to die. "We will drain your blood, drop by drop. When half the blood drops, you will go into a coma and just die." They made a small prick in his skin. Then, they opened the tap of a tank and let the water drip into a bucket. After a few minutes, the prisoner became paler and paler and died.

Similarly, you believe that you are living, so you live. You believe that you are dying, so you die. In reality, we are the unchanging, never-dying principle. This is not just a false suggestion. What you are suggesting is in fact the falsehood. When you talk in terms of your body and mind, then that is falsehood. For example, you say you are sitting. You are lying. The body is sitting. In the name of spirituality, we are asked to think in the name of truth. Regarding these yogic teachings, Yoga is not another religion. Yoga embodies the basic principles that are in every religion. Wherever you see the foundation of any religion, you see the yogic principle. The way you sit and worship may vary, but the common requisites don't vary.

Question: Although nothing is really evil, don't we have to practice renunciation?

Sri Gurudev: If you are not renounced, even the so-called good things become evil. A renounced person will feel, "Nothing is mine" or "All is mine," because he or she is not attached to anything. It's not as though renounced people are indifferent to things. Rather, it is the personal attachment to those things that they renounce.

In the beginning, we need to be in a protected environment. When spiritual feelings come as a small flame, we need the company of those who can help us kindle that flame. If you want to follow a particular path, you must also follow those associated with that path.

OM Shanthi, Shanthi, Shanthi.

Chapter 4
The Art of Giving and Receiving

Usually, selfless service melts even the hardest hearts.

—Sri Swami Satchidananda

Teaching Yoga—or, for that matter, any other subject—in prison offers both students and instructors a fantastic opportunity to develop unconditional love. Of course, that opportunity presents itself to us everywhere, 24/7. But the charged atmosphere of prison forces us to come to terms with our own heavy baggage in the form of hidden fears and secret prejudices, pre-conceived notions and suppressed anxieties. In this particular setting, we are unambiguously confronted with our strengths and weaknesses. What's more, we discover a connection: We are all in pursuit of happiness. We come to realize that most people who end up in prison are there because, just like us, they are searching for happiness.

Yes, we all want to be happy. And we all want to be free. In fact, the most famous statement in the Declaration of Independence of the United States lists three aspects among the inalienable rights of human beings: life, liberty and the pursuit of happiness. Ironically, the US currently incarcerates more people than any other country in the world. Why? On the personal level, the answer correlates to the following questions. How do we live our lives? In what manner do we make use of our liberty? And by what means do we pursue our happiness? Put simply, are we living productively or destructively? Do we behave selflessly or selfishly? Do our actions bring benefit or harm others? Obviously, these questions are rhetorical and the answers are self-evident. As Gurudev used to say, when our life, liberty and pursuit of happiness are permeated with destructive acts that arise from selfish desires, we exchange freedom for free-dumb. In this case, some of us end up in prison, maybe even on Death Row.

Even if most of us don't wind up in prison, it's probably safe to say that we have all suffered from a variety of selfish desires that sometimes motivate us to hurt others, as well as ourselves, in one way or another; in this sense, to some degree, we have something in common with people who are doing time in prison. As to my own misdeeds, I remember at least one incident that I'm not so proud of.

When I was about twelve or thirteen years old, I discovered that some of my friends were stealing lipsticks from a large five-and-dime store and cheap costume jewelry from a flea market in the city. One day, they invited me along. I don't know whether they stole because they had no money to pay for the items or because they enjoyed the thrill; I did it because I wanted to belong; and, I must admit, there was something exciting about breaking the rules. I was involved in a couple of these capers, but my conscience finally got the better of me. None of us ever got caught. Luckily, for my friends and me, and for everyone else in our lives, the thrill of breaking the law wore off. We reformed. Having had at least a taste of what it feels like to commit a crime, though a petty one, what came to mind when I began volunteering at the Buckingham Correction center was: there but for the grace of God go I. As Bo Lozoff, who founded the Ashram Prison Project, wrote: "We're all doing time."

Yes, we're all prisoners: prisoners of our concepts, our prejudices, our habits, our beliefs, our desires, our ego, our ignorance. But as in all prisons, there's a key that opens the door to freedom. The key that will release us from our inner prison is self-knowledge. For when we experience the reality that we are more than the body and mind, that we are not separated from anyone or anything in the universe, and that our perceived limitations are self-imposed, then we will know the joy of real freedom. The teachings and practices of Yoga have been utilized for thousands of years by those who long to be liberated, to experience the unity of being, to realize the true Self. In fact, all the branches of Yoga* lead us to liberation from the machinations of our mischievous egos by helping us refine the body and the mind and by deepening our spiritual awareness.

---

* (Karma Yoga, the path of selfless service; Jnana Yoga, the path of self-inquiry; Hatha Yoga, the path of physical refinement through postures and breath control; Bhakti Yoga, the path of devotion; Japa Yoga, repetition of a mantra, or sacred sound; and Raja Yoga, the path of mastery of the mind through meditation.)

The Integral Yoga teachers who have brought, and who are still bringing, Yoga into prison are trained in all these branches of Yoga. To give you a taste of what some of these individuals have encountered, this chapter will introduce you to some of them.

Sudharman Joseph Fenton

Sudharman Fenton, who served in the military as a Navy Seal, currently directs an Integral Yoga Center in New Berlin, Pennsylvania. He began teaching Integral Yoga in Virginia state and federal prisons in the early 1970s. His prison experience is unique.

Right after taking a ten-day silent retreat, Sudharman visited a prison where his brother was the warden. During the visit, Sudharman's brother talked about various problems that he saw in the prisons, also discussing his solutions to these predicaments. At the time, Sudharman was living at Satchidananda Ashram-Yogaville in Buckingham, Virginia, and when he returned to the *ashram*, he thought for a long time about the conversation he'd had with his brother regarding prison issues. Then, when the time came for him to leave the *ashram*, he had a plan. He decided to open a prison with his brother. His brother would run the prison, and Sudharman would teach Yoga there. The plan actually did come to fruition and for several years Sudharman and his brother owned and operated a private prison.

Sudharman told me that up to 80 percent of inmates across the US have drug or alcohol issues and that, often, it's drug addiction that keeps them in prison. Obviously, drug rehabilitation programs would benefit this population. Also, such programs would help to alleviate some of the enormous expense of maintaining prisoners. However, according to Sudharman, and from my own experience as a prison teacher, attitudes regarding prison rehabilitation programs (including college degree programs) change, because they are contingent upon whether the state administration happens to be liberal or conservative: conservative officials tend not to be in favor of providing such programs, while liberal administrators usually support them.

Moreover, the frequent elimination of programs and changes of attitudes with respect to what types of activities foster rehabilitation play havoc with prisoner and staff morale: the staff becomes almost schizophrenic from continually having to adapt to opposing attitudes, and the prisoners lose morale when they are deprived of programs that broaden their awareness, offer them skills that will give them more opportunity to make a living when they leave prison, increase their self-confidence and keep their minds active in positive ways.

In Sudharman's experience, the many prisoners who want to study and practice Yoga are sincere. He really enjoyed working with them. Sudharman found that while "almost nothing works well in prison, Yoga does."

Rev. Jaganath Carrera

Rev. Jaganath Carrera is an Integral Yoga minister who has been teaching Yoga for many years in New Jersey and served for several years as an administrator at Satchidananda Ashram. He is the author of *Inside the Yoga Sutras: A Sourcebook for the Study and Practice of Patanjali's Yoga Sutras* and the director of the Yoga Life Society.

For more than three years, during the 70s, Rev. Jaganath taught Yoga at Trenton State Prison, a maximum security prison in Trenton, New Jersey. He had already been teaching Integral Yoga for several years, but it had never occurred to him to teach in prison until a friend approached him. The friend, a psychologist who, himself, practiced Yoga, was interested in having Yoga taught at the college where he was working and he asked Jaganath whether he'd be interested. Jaganath agreed to teach there and he waited for his friend to contact him. However, when his friend finally did call, it was to tell Jaganath that it hadn't worked out at the college and that, instead, he had found him a job teaching Yoga at a nearby prison. Jaganath was soon hired by the State of New Jersey to teach Yoga in prison.

In a talk about prison Yoga that he gave at the *ashram* to students of the Basic *Hatha* Teaching Training, Rev. Jaganath emphasized the following two requirements for those who were interested in teaching Yoga in prisons: (1) complete honesty when interacting with students, and (2) the understanding that you are there to serve rather than to help students. He went on to describe the intimidating atmosphere that he encountered at the beginning of his tenure at Trenton State Prison.

The first time he went to the prison, he drove down the wrong road, so he stopped to ask a guard for help. The guard had a shotgun which he held near the car window while he waited for Jaganath to say what he had to say; then, the guard led Jaganath to the right building. Once inside the building, Jaganath was frisked twice, once with a metal detector and once hands-on. He was told that if he was at all late when he came to teach, he wouldn't be allowed in.

The atmosphere was charged—approximately 67 percent of the men were convicted of murder and 28 percent were convicted of rape. Also, there had been recent hostility over religious differences, and there were racial issues. Furthermore, Jaganath found that the prisoners' perception was that they hadn't been treated fairly or given a fair chance in life, so, feeling disadvantaged, they would do whatever they needed to do to protect themselves.

Additionally, the physical environment was dismal. The buildings were terribly dilapidated. There was one guard for an entire wing. There were twenty-two men in the class and no guard in the classroom. The men entered the classroom by wing and they left the two-hour session in the same way, wing by wing.

Jaganath walked into the first class, sat down and waited for the men to come in. Some men were smoking and the first thing that Jaganath said was: "Stop smoking. During this class, there will be no smoking." Then, he told them: "I'm not here to help you. It doesn't matter to me whether you come or not. I'm here to be used, not abused." Also, he gave them the ground rules: no smoking, no foul language, no mumbling. And this clicked with the men.

All the men who came to the Yoga class volunteered to come. And since it was the only way that they could get out of their cells at night, they really wanted to be there.

Jaganath told the following story. One of the inmates in the class sat not far from Jaganath every week. This man had huge muscles, a shaved head and gold teeth. According to Jaganath, he looked life-threatening. This prisoner was called Mr. Smart. Mr.

Smart spent the entire class glaring at Jaganath with cold eyes and he didn't do any of the Yoga postures. Jaganath considered it a possibility that Mr. Smart might jump up and attack him. This went on for five or six weeks. One day, Jaganath decided to cut the *Hatha* class short in order to include a longer meditation and a talk about meditation. At this point, he felt that something special was happening with the group; there seemed to be a special atmosphere in the room, a feeling of peace. The meditation session lasted for about forty-five minutes, and when the guard announced that the class was over, Jaganath noticed that Mr. Smart had tears rolling out of his eyes. He nudged Jaganath and said, "Thank you." After that class, everything changed. Jaganath thought that maybe Mr. Smart had been the leader of the group. In any case, Mr. Smart did become the leader in that class. He started doing *Hatha* every day on his bed, because there was no room on the cell floor; he meditated; he read Yoga books; and he became the disciplinarian in the class. Eventually, Mr. Smart was released from prison, and he took a job as a school janitor in Florida.

The *Hatha* class took place once a week during the regular forty-two week school term. It wasn't too long before Jaganath noticed remarkable changes in the men. In fact, eventually the warden called him to say that the men who were taking Yoga classes were showing marked improvement in their jobs. The warden even offered to get anything that Jaganath wanted for the course, so Jaganath ordered copies of the *Yoga Sutras of Patanjali* (the essential text of the philosophy and practices of Yoga), pens and pencils and carpeting. What's more, he started teaching three days a week and was asked to increase his classes to five days a week, as well as evenings. The men were interested in *Raja Yoga*, so he taught a forty-two week *Raja Yoga* class. In fact, he had to keep creating different Yoga courses, as each course was filled up and there were waiting lists.

Another vital point that Jaganath brought up about teaching in prison is that inmates will test the instructor in various ways. If you preach about peace, for instance, they'll test your peace. If you tell them that peace lies within us all or that peace is our true nature, then you'd better have faith in your convictions. And if you say that you'll do something, do it. This is a tremendous practice for the teacher, too, because prisoners are always testing your authenticity, and it takes a long time to gain their trust.

According to what was happening in the prison, Jaganath made changes in the course. One day, a new rule was put into effect: all visitors, including family members, had to be strip-searched, and the search included all orifices, because drugs and weapons were being smuggled in. So that week, instead of teaching the usual Yoga class, Jaganath facilitated a two-hour conversation where the men expressed their feelings about the situation; addressing the issue in a group discussion helped them to take a rational, more objective view of the situation.

Sadly, some inmates had known only institutional life for almost their whole lives and were not able to function outside prison. Most men in Trenton State Prison were in for life or had an average 30-year sentence. Some men sat in their cells all day long, going out to the yard only once a day. Furthermore, their diet was *tamasic* (a Sanskrit term that refers to the quality of sluggishness): mostly starchy foods and no fresh vegetables except for iceberg lettuce; only on weekends were they served lemons, oranges and bananas. The result was that they were constipated and often suffered from hemorrhoids. In such a situation, Jaganath said, the Yoga teacher could offer valuable advice about diet and nutrition, so that the inmates could, at least sometimes, make good choices.

Along with this description of his own prison teaching experience and his advice to teachers who might consider teaching in prison, Jaganath shared some inspiring anecdotes.

One inmate loved Sri Gurudev, whom he'd met only through books and whom he called "The Sage." He even made a drawing of Gurudev, which he gave to Jaganath as a gift. One day, he was meditating on his bed in front of Gurudev's book on the *Yoga Sutras* when he had a vision of a rainbow coming out of the faucet in the sink that was in his cell. The rainbow went up and down, spreading out like a fountain. On the top of the rainbow, where it crested, was an image of Mother Mary, and he knew that the Mother was with him. He drew a picture of this vision. This fellow did get out of prison and took a job as a computer programmer.

Toward the end of Jaganath's tenure at Trenton State Prison, a stirring poem by Sri Swami Vivekananda about the liberating power of renunciation was put to music. Swami Vivekananda was a renowned sage from India and, in 1893, he was the first swami to visit the United States. The poem, entitled "Song of the Free," was set to music and was sung and recorded by an American Integral Yoga swami who was also called Swami Vivekananda. One day, Jaganath brought the poem to class. The men loved it, reading it over and over again. So Jaganath brought the taped musical version. As they listened to the tape, the men began to sing along with it. They played the tape several times, singing along with it, and each time they played the tape, their voices got louder and louder. Finally, when they stopped playing the tape, they heard the guys in the cells outside the room yelling, "Do it again!" This event occurred during the last class that Jaganath taught at the prison.

Prakash Shakti Capen

Prakash Shakti Capen, a resident of Yogaville, served at the *ashram* and at several Integral Yoga Institutes on both US coasts. For a number of years, she edited the *Integral Yoga Magazine* and managed Integral Yoga Publications. In the late 1970s, she taught Yoga in two Boston prisons. Prakash became involved in prison Yoga when a prison official contacted the Integral Yoga Institute in Boston, where Prakash was living at the time, because she was interested in introducing Yoga into prisons in the greater Boston area. Prakash worked with this woman on a proposal, which was turned down the first time it was submitted. However, the official didn't give up, and her proposal was finally accepted.

Before Prakash began teaching in the prisons, the official took her and some others on a tour of a maximum-security and a minimum-security prison for men. Prakash remembered that during the visits, prisoners were yelling up to her from the yard. As a woman, she felt pretty vulnerable. Indeed, her first prison class presented quite a challenge. While Prakash discussed Yoga, all the men talked with each other and some smoked. When Prakash asked them to stop talking and smoking, they grumbled. Little by little, though, Prakash and her students established a good rapport, and the discussions became meaningful. In fact, when one of the men, a gruff fellow, came late to one class, smoking a cigarette, the other guys said, "Put it out—now!" At this point, the men were beginning to bond with Prakash and with each other.

Prakash also recalled that during the first class, the men refused to close their eyes in *savaasana* (the "corpse pose"), the relaxation pose. They remained still and looked relaxed, but they wouldn't close their eyes. However, when Prakash asked them to sit up to do the breathing practices, they all sat up and automatically, without any direction, closed their eyes.

Many of the men continued in the class. They were always interested in how Yoga could bring them power. And while they wanted to learn how Yoga could help them become centered, they were always focused on how, through Yoga, they could acquire *siddhis*, or powers, that would render them invincible. Prakash explained that although certain attainments could be gained as a result of the yogic practices, the goal of Yoga is not to attain powers but to become easeful, peaceful and useful human beings. On the positive side, Prakash saw that their interest in achieving yogic powers did motivate them to do *pranayama*, the breathing practices, regularly and enthusiastically, She helped them develop their practice slowly and carefully, explaining that if they practiced *pranayama* excessively when the body and mind were not ready, that is, if the nervous system is not strong and the mind is not balanced, they could bring harm to both the body and the mind.

Apparently, the inmates' enthusiasm for Yoga was contagious, because, sometimes, even the guard would join, doing some of the postures and *Yoga Nidra*, deep relaxation. Once, in fact, he went so deeply into deep relaxation that he didn't wake up when the signal was given. So, while all the inmates were sitting up, he was still lying on the floor—with his gun on his hip. The men simply smiled.

A fitting testament to the power of Yoga, to its efficacy in prison, and surely, to the peaceful vibe (and probably the faith) of Prakash, who was delighted to see the fully relaxed guard awaken only when the men began the closing chants at the end of the class.

Swami Karunananda Ma

Swami Karunananda, one of Integral Yoga's principal teachers, developed, and leads, Raja Yoga and Meditation Teacher Training courses and workshops. She has served as the director of the San Francisco and Santa Barbara Integral Yoga Institutes and as president of Satchidananda Ashram-Yogaville. For a number of months, in the mid-1970s, she and another Integral Yoga teacher, Bhaktan Eberle, taught at the San Francisco County jail. Bhaktan went to the men's jail and Swami Karunananda to the women's.

One of the challenges that Karunananda Ma recalls is that in this prison there was no dedicated space available where she could hold a Yoga class, so the class had to be held in a common area where inmates watched TV.

Swami Karunananda also taught a few times at San Bruno, another prison in the San Francisco area. She remembers going through gate after gate; one gate would slam closed behind her and one would open in front of her, door after door, from building to building. And she also remembers an unusual experience:

The class was very big and the students were both male and female, with many young people attending. There must have been a couple of hundred inmates in the class, but Swami Karunananda didn't see a single guard. At first, all the students stood in front of her. Then, they circled around her. And as she spoke, they began closing in on her. Was there an unspoken agreement among them? In any case, no one intervened. So, she just kept talking as though nothing unusual were happening. Even though she felt cocooned in a tight circle, she appeared calm. She must have passed some sort of test because at a certain point the circle began to widen, she gave her introduction to Yoga and then, taught the class.

A strange occurrence, perhaps, but Karunananda wondered

whether it might have been the karmic result of a previous experience that took place many, many years before when she was in elementary school. She remembered that once, for a week, her class had a substitute teacher. None of the students liked this teacher, so they pulled a prank. Every time the teacher turned around to write on the board, the kids moved their desks a few inches closer to the teacher, creeping up toward her, little by little, during the 45 minutes of class. At some point, when the teacher turned back to face the class, she was surrounded by a tiny, tight circle, which she found really disturbing.

The law of *karma* manifests in mysterious ways.

Vimala Nora Pozzi

Vimala Nora Pozzi, director of the Integral Yoga Institute of Richmond, Virginia, organized a prison project in 1998. As part of this project, ten to fifteen teachers and advanced students began teaching Yoga at the Bon Air Juvenile Correctional Center, a juvenile detention center in the Richmond area. Vimala and the other Integral Yoga instructors had been teaching at the facility for two years, offering classes twice a week to the girls housed in the center. During this program, the instructors went to the girls' cottages. One of the challenges was the great turnover of students. The program was not compulsory, so teachers never knew from one class to another who, and how many, would be attending. Consequently, Vimala felt that this was a great opportunity not only for the girls to learn Yoga, but also for the instructors to practice non-attachment.

As Vimala describes it, there were a number of challenges that came with teaching in a juvenile correctional center, including many distractions during classes, which were held in the gym: bathroom trips required a guard as an escort, the PA system sounded announcements, girls were called out of class to go to special meetings or counseling, and girls from other classrooms walked through the gym. In such a distracting environment, the goal of the Yoga instructors was to use Yoga as a technique to help the girls focus the mind and concentrate in the midst of activity. Vimala, herself, found that in order to teach in such an environment, she needed some special tools: patience, mindfulness, a non-judgmental attitude, compassion, flexibility, open-mindedness and creativity. Additionally, she told stories, used visualization, led meditations on positive and negative emotions and encouraged the girls to become introspective.

In the Summer 2000 issue of *The OM News*, a newsletter published by the Integral Yoga Institute of Richmond, Vimala printed a few of the thank you letters that she received from her Yoga students at the Bon Air Juvenile Correctional Center. The two that follow echo the positive sentiments expressed by many of the girls:

> Ms. Pozzi, this class has helped me to work out my emotional as well as physical problems. You have also helped me in ways you would never imagine. My favorite pose is the Tree Pose, but my favorite thing about Yoga is deep relaxation. Thank you for coming, and I hope to see you again.

> Ms. Pozzi,

> I would like to thank you for coming here and for teaching us to do Yoga. You have helped me a great deal. I must admit, I have an anger problem, and you have taught me the deep relaxation techniques that helped me a lot. I was not really excited to do Yoga when you first came. But then you started talking about the history of it, and it seemed very interesting, so I decided to try. I am not very good at it, but you inspired me not to give up and to try again. You have helped me a great deal with my problems and with a lot of my stress, and I greatly appreciate it.

> One of my most favorite stretches is the Cobra Pose. It not only releases stress, but also relieves the pain in my lower back, as well as strengthens my upper body. If you ever find the time and patience, we would be very grateful for you to come back and teach us some more Yoga. I know that I, myself, plan on taking many more Yoga classes and hope to get very good at it.

Bhavani Kludt and Donnelle Malnik

Bhavani Kludt, an Integral Yoga-trained instructor from the San Francisco area, founded a prison program called RSVP (Resolve to Stop the Violence). The premise of RSVP is that many people who are incarcerated are filled with self-hatred that they project onto others. The focus of this program, which Bhavani developed in order to help people work through the reasons for their self-hatred and violent behavior, is based on the principle of *ahimsa*, or non-violence, the first of the ten *yama/niyama** (moral and ethical principles listed in Patanjali's *Yoga Sutras)*. Utilizing Yoga to explore their inner world, inmates begin to understand and to nurture themselves. As they come to love and respect themselves, they develop compassion and respect for others.

To ensure that the RSVP program reached as many inmates as possible, Bhavani has trained several teachers. Donnelle Malnik is one of them, and in a video entitled *Going Within*, she gives us a glimpse of the program and her involvement in it.

Donnelle feels deeply that prisoners deserve an opportunity to transform their lives, and she believes that her own challenging background gives her special insight into the experiences and suffering of many of those who end up in prison. Like many people who are incarcerated, Donnelle came from a completely dysfunctional family. She had a harsh childhood, or, as she puts it, really no childhood at all. Brought up in an abusive environment, she had to fend for herself at an early age.

In the video, Donnelle talks about some of the participants in the RSVP program, describing their experiences and insights. One man, who became partially paralyzed after being shot, said that he came to realize that he was always afraid to live. On the physical level, he felt that Yoga was helping him more than physical therapy. Another prisoner stated that, through meditation, he was learning to release negativity and to feel peace, while someone

---

*Yama: *non-violence, truthfulness, non-stealing, continence and non-greed.* Niyama: *purity, contentment, accepting but not causing pain, study of spiritual books, and worship of God [self-surrender].*

else remarked that the open discussion, which was part of their meditation process, was helping him reduce stress and overcome depression. Then there was the student who was deeply affected by the deep breathing practices. As he recounted it, his heart opened up when he realized that everyone shares the same oxygen and that we all just want to be happy. Finally, one participant summed up his experience: the Yoga made him aware of good things.

As for Donnelle, facilitating this program has led her to the realization that prison inmates are, like all of us, survivors who want to be happy. She came to see these individuals as human beings. And she feels quite strongly that if inmates are not offered programs like RSVP, which focus on self-awareness and self-reformation, then, when they are released from prison, it won't be long before they repeat their old negative patterns and find themselves back in prison.

Chapter 5
Freedom Begins at *OM*

Teach me to feel another's woe, To hide the fault I see.
That mercy I to others show,
That mercy show to me.

—Alexander Pope (The Universal Prayer, Stanza 10)

According to a new report released on February 14, 2007, by the Public Safety Performance Project of The Pew Charitable Trusts, by 2011, one in every 178 residents of the United States of America will live in prison. A recent online BBC News article reported that, according to government figures, the number of people incarcerated in the US rose to more than two million, indicating that the US has the largest prison population in the world, as well as the highest number of inmates in proportion to its population. Moreover, as the article states, that figure would be higher if inmates handled by the US Immigration and Naturalization Service, and those in military jails and other institutions, were included. *Confronting Confinement*, a study undertaken in June 2006 by the bipartisan Commission on Safety and Abuse in America's Prisons, reports that over the course of a year, 13.5 million individuals spend time in prison or jail.

It should also be noted that one doesn't have to be an expert to recognize that in the United States, stress-related illnesses—mental problems, hypertension, stroke, heart disease, cancer and autoimmune diseases—are on the rise and that unrelieved stress plays a big part in crime, drug abuse and domestic violence. Americans are suffering from stress inside and outside of prisons. Of course, there's no simple solution to any of these complex issues. However, as this book illustrates, Yoga has proven itself, through the ages and in diverse settings, to be an efficacious method of managing stress and enhancing physical and mental health and well being. In fact, these days, a growing number of prison personnel are becoming aware of Yoga and its potential to alleviate the stress that permeates the lives of prison inmates and prison staff alike. According to some reports, a huge number of inmates are released back into society, but, sadly, a large percentage of those are re-arrested and re-incarcerated. It's my conviction, from my own experience as a prison volunteer and from the experience of other volunteers that Yoga can and does play a part in lowering the recidivism rate by helping inmates develop positive and creative thinking, making them better equipped when they are released to face life's challenges with a more positive self-image, with greater self-confidence. I hope that more and more prisons will make Yoga programs available to inmates and that more and more Yoga teachers will make themselves available as prison volunteers. I am happy to report that, currently, there are several highly effective prison Yoga programs already working their wonders, nationally and internationally.

Bo Lozoff's Prison-Ashram Project

No doubt, the most well-known proponent of Yoga in prison is Bo Lozoff, author of *We're All Doing Time, A Guide for Getting Free*. In the early 70s, Lozoff visited some friends who were imprisoned, without possibility of parole, for smuggling marijuana into Miami. Distressed by their anguish and by conditions in the prison, he felt an overwhelming urge to do something. He applied for a job at the prison but was turned down. However, an assistant warden, intrigued by Lozoff's idea of offering Yoga and meditation instruction to prisoners, suggested that Lozoff submit a proposal to federal authorities, and Lozoff did just that. The authorities went for the idea. Lozoff was flown to Washington to be interviewed at the Bureau of Prisons. He was hired as a consultant, was given permission to offer classes in federal institutions and was invited to conduct Prison-Ashram classes and workshops in the US and abroad. Additionally, Lozoff and his wife, Sita, sent thousands of letters, books and tapes to inquiring inmates, their families, prison workers, veterans, the handicapped and anyone else who was interested. But I'm jumping ahead of myself. To backtrack and to give you a sense of Lozoff's passion, his spiritual perspective, his sense of purpose and commitment to serving the prison population and to service in general, I'd like to share with you some excerpts from an interview that appeared in the Spring 2008 issue of *Integral Yoga Magazine*.

"Prison Yoga: We're All Doing Time"
An Interview with Bo Lozoff

Integral Yoga Magazine: How did you get into Yoga?

Bo Lozoff: My first Yoga class was with Swami Satchidananda in 1972 at the University of North Carolina, Chapel Hill. There were 200 people in shoulder stand, and he's walking in and out of the rows of students, and our two-year-old son is walking next to him like an assistant! I first started veering toward Yoga in the early 1970s when I got a job in psychic research at Duke. I was the point man for yogis and swamis for the Psychical Research foundation on the campus of Duke. Gurudev came down for an experiment when I was there. A local devotee also participated. We put them in two separate rooms and wired them to EEG machines which measure brain waves. We showed Gurudev different photos–nice things, harsh things–to see if his devotee, who was trying to tune into him, would have a parallel EEG. The results were mildly significant, showing some correlation. Eventually, I left, because I was more moved by the swamis whom we tested than by the science. So, I took a few classes from Gurudev. My 20-minute *Hatha* routine is based on what I learned from him. I'm not trying to become an advanced *Hatha* Yogi; I'm, basically, a *Karma Yogi*.

IYM: How did the Prison Ashram Project start?

BL: In 1972, somebody gave my wife, Sita, a copy of *Be Here Now* by Ram Dass, which she recommended that I also read. When I opened it, the first page was a photo of Neem Karoli Baba (Maharaj-ji), Ram Dass's guru. I recognized him as the "magic man" about whom I had begun dreaming when I was eight years old. That got my attention! I must have dreamt of him a hundred times or more. I never could have imagined that he was real. I was 25 when I finally saw a photo of him and his face was more familiar to me than my own. Within a short time, I was a fulltime yogi. We wrote to Ram Dass, and he visited us in 1973, and we became instantly connected. We talked about doing a prison *ashram* project . . . I had no context for what I wanted to do in the prisons. We went to the Federal Bureau of Prisons to discuss the idea of offering classes. At the time that I talked with Ram Dass about it, he was beginning to get correspondence from prisoners, since they were reading his book, *Be Here Now*. He offered me some postage money to answer the letters. Letters started to pour in. We never planned to create a lifelong prison ministry, but that's what happened. We just quietly started sending free books and writing to people.

IYM: So, what are you doing now?

BL: My life tends to run in tides of going inward and going outward. Every ten years or so, I do retreats. In 2001, I did a year of silence. After my tour ended in 2007, I decided not to do public speaking or teaching in 2008. [Lozoff had recently completed a 22-month prison tour, visiting 300 prisons, Yoga centers and churches, giving hundreds of workshops.] I'm now going into silence and rejuvenating my singing career, which was put on the back burner . . . . When I went into silence in 2001, I didn't miss talking, but I really missed chanting and singing.

IYM: What do you talk about to the prisoners?

BL: The only thing I feel that I have to share is my seriousness about the spiritual journey. I have nothing to sell, no philosophy, no teachings to give, no special path. What I do and what I encourage others to do is to go deep on their own spiritual path and journey. I haven't created Integral Yoga or *Vipassana* . . . I'm me, so I have to follow that journey. My tide goes inward and outward. I think [all individuals are] doing what they feel is right for them. When I went into silence in 2001 and I told my mother that I wasn't going to speak to her for a year, her reaction was, "You are 55-years-old and you have done so much good; why can't you just relax and have a good time?" I said, "You're right, mom, but I'm hardwired to do these things."

I'd hesitate to give any formula for how someone can translate idealism into service. I've given away hundreds of thousands of dollars, homes and copyrights, not because I think that everyone should do that, but because I'm disinterested in material security. I don't want to know that I will be taken care of or be okay. To me, life is a daredevil adventure. People offer me all kinds of things, but the fun in life is living according to your beliefs, doing what you feel is right and taking what comes. If you want to be a heart surgeon, you will probably become wealthy. If your genuine interest is to be a songwriter, you'll probably be poor. It doesn't matter. Follow the energy and take the adventure.

IYM: How do you find balance between taking care of yourself and service?

BL: For me there is no balance. No matter how eloquently you phrase it, what we are really talking about in regard to balance is about me vs. service. I think that is a flawed perspective. My life is meaningless if I'm not of service. I have people tell me all the time, "Take some 'Bo time.' You do so much for others; you'd better get a massage; take a break; take time for yourself." It seems almost a vicious attack against service! I don't live in a world where my service is martyring me. I live in a world where I don't serve well enough. I have friends who have fallen into a world where they change the words of the song, "Amazing Grace," to be politically correct. They sing: "To save a soul like me" [instead of "To save a wretch like me"]. What should we be looking for: mediocre, reasonable grace, how sweet it is? I deal with wretches–people who have killed and raped but who are worthy of grace. It wouldn't be amazing grace if it was about a parking ticket!

IYM: Is there something wrong with taking care of ourselves as we serve?

BL: There's too much apprehension about doing *seva* and worrying about security issues. When you worry about giving too much away, you're missing the point. Just be careful when you think that your service is a big deal. I'm doing what I'm inclined to do, and I'm not sure that I'm doing my *seva* well enough, but I'm doing what I can. Yoga and all wisdom paths tell us that our needs are met when we give it all away. I don't want the apprehension that comes with worrying about my well being. When you accept the core spiritual principle that you are gonna be sliced, diced and crucified, that no one gets out alive, when you accept that you are perishing as you speak, then everything falls into perspective. Service isn't something to take care of when you get everything you want. Service is why you are here.

IYM: You don't feel the need to take care of yourself at all?

BL: The way I take care of Bo is to take care of others. I don't see any merit to cautious ideas of moderation and making sure we take care of ourselves when our planet is dying. Let's have a great time serving others and understanding *tikkun*, the Hebrew word for "world repair." We are here to serve, to repair the world. This is *seva*, this is what we are to be dedicated to ... Yes, I need to do my Yoga, to eat right and so on, but not because it's "me time." That's what I don't like about pop culture spirituality. It takes everything and puts it in service of the egoistic self. That doesn't work. That self will never get all it wants. That self has to die.

When people live in the kind of context that my altar has to be set up just so, I need to *feng shui* my house or I can't live there, I have to be comfortable, feel good, they can become very uptight. I think that being a spiritual seeker means to become a humbler, quieter and more tolerant individual when we live in a place where it doesn't all go our way. If you read all the spiritual books, do all the spiritual practices that you're supposed to, how long does any unblemished period last before life intrudes and brings something very unwelcome? When I walk into a maximum-security prison, I had better find out if there is still anything good, if life is still worth living, and if I can't find it, then I'm of no service to those prisoners ... I trust service, I trust life and I don't have a sense that this work has to go on, that it's so important. I know what I'm inclined to offer; but how useful or selfless my service is, that's for others to decide ... What I find lacking in American spirituality is humility. The most inspiring people like Swami Chidanandaji [Divine Life Society, Rishikesh, India] and Swami Satchidanandaji are incredibly humble people.

With Ram Dass, Bo and Sita Lozoff founded the largest prison interfaith ministry in the world. This ministry serves in 60 countries, with 50,000 prisoners on its mailing list. *We're All Doing Time*, now in its seventeenth printing (half a million copies have been distributed thus far), is referred to as the "prisoners' bible." A prison classic, it is provided free to anyone in prison and to others who can't afford to pay for it. "Book One" discusses the challenges of living a fulfilling life no matter what one's circumstances are, the law of *karma* and non-attachment. "Book Two" offers various practices that can help one achieve spiritual awareness–meditation, *Hatha Yoga*, *pranayama* and proper diet, prayer and *Karma Yoga*, or selfless service. And "Book Three" consists of letters. All proceeds from the sale of the book go toward supporting this free distribution. To receive a copy of the book, write to: Human Kindness Foundation: PO Box 61619, Durham, North Carolina 27715.

Siddha Yoga Prison Project

In its November/December 2006 Online Extra issue, *Yoga Journal* included an article about the Siddha Yoga Prison Project, a 25-year-old non-profit program that has offered free Yoga instruction through correspondence courses to at least 45,000 prisoners worldwide. The largest program of its kind in the United States, Siddha Yoga Project provides more than 6,000 inmates in 1,200 prisons with Yoga classes and monthly newsletters.

Featured in the article, "A New Conviction," by Jaimal Yogis, is an interview with Ted Hyde, an Account Executive, who volunteers with the Siddha Yoga Prison Project. A former prisoner who was released a few years ago from a California state prison, Hyde acknowledges that Yoga helped him to get his life back together. Moreover, he credits Siddha Yoga for his successful reentry into society. He recounts that when he was released from prison, the local Siddha Yoga center invited him to take free classes, which he started taking right away. The sense of community proved crucial to him, especially because his wife had left him while he was in prison.

Now, Ted Hyde is returning to prison, not as a prisoner, but as a volunteer who serves his community by teaching Yoga and meditation. He told his interviewer, "When I walked out of prison and those doors closed behind me, I thought I would never want to go back inside. But I can be of help now. I know this works."

Insight Prison Project

The Insight Prison Project (IPP), created in 1998, is dedicated to creating and conducting effective rehabilitation programs inside prison. IPP is a non-profit community organization that works in collaboration with San Quentin State Prison in San Rafael, California. According to its web site, "the key to IPP's success has been its extraordinary group of facilitators, who are dedicated to creating positive change both inside and outside the prison walls." IPP includes professional counseling and therapy, conflict resolution and mediation, 12-step programs, victim/offender dialogues, violence prevention, anger management training, pre-parole planning, gardening and landscaping, Yoga instruction and meditation.

In partnership with San Quentin State Prison, IPP offers eighteen unique programs each week, serving approximately 300 inmates. The majority of IPP's classes take place as part of the STAND UP Program, for which IPP is the largest program provider.

STAND UP Program

STAND UP, initiated by San Quentin's Warden Bob Ayers, is a collaboration between the prison and a variety of organizations whose goal is to offer academic, vocational, self-development and post-release services to prisoners. STAND UP succeeds the Success Program, which IPP helped to initiate in 2002. The Success Program provided some 200,000 individual hours of education and self-development in four and a half years. Former warden, Jeanne Woodford, launched the program during her tenure at San Quentin. In an interview with *Yoga Journal*, Woodford explained that she had incorporated Yoga into the program because she felt that it was important to offer inmates different ways of looking at the world so that they might make better life choices. She felt that Yoga was an excellent tool in this regard because it teaches self-discipline and an understanding of body, mind and soul. Moreover, she was encouraged by the success of the meditation program at the San Francisco County Jail and similar programs in India.

The Prison Dharma Network

The Prison Dharma Network (PDN), headquartered in Boulder, Colorado, is an international, non-sectarian contemplative support network for prisoners, prison volunteers and corrections professionals. PDN's mission is to provide prisoners, as well as those who work with prisoners, the most effective contemplative methods for self-transformation and rehabilitation. Staff members lead Yoga and meditation sessions in prisons and correspond with and send books to thousands of prisoners nationwide. Emphasis is on sitting meditation practice and the practice and study of Buddhist teachings and other wisdom traditions. PDN promotes the paths of wakefulness and non-aggression, which it views as ideal vehicles for self-rehabilitation and personal transformation.

Prison Dharma Network was founded in 1985 by Fleet Maull, not long after he was incarcerated on drug charges. Prior to his incarceration, Maull had received extensive training as a meditation instructor under the guidance of well-known Tibetan meditation master, Chogyam Trungpa Rinpoche. He directed PDN for twelve years from inside the prison with the help of outside volunteers. During his fourteen years in prison (he was released in 1999), Fleet Maull also helped to start the first prison hospice program. Today, there are over twenty hospice programs in state and federal facilities across the country. Fleet Maull is the author of *Dharma in Hell: The Prison Writings of Fleet Maull*, and he is the subject of Roshi Bernie Glassman's book, *Bearing Witness*.

Like all those who support and participate in transformational prison rehabilitation programs, PDN values "the healing and transformational paradigm of the Restorative and Transformative models of criminal justice practice over the more punitive paradigm of Retributive Justice models."

Freeing the Human Spirit

Freeing the Human Spirit, a British prison program that has attracted the support of actor Jeremy Irons, "helps prisoners deal with their anger and stay out of jail through the practice of Yoga and meditation." In an article that appeared on the website, www.ctv.ca, Irons acknowledges that his work as an actor enabled him to connect with prisoners. Irons told CTV's Canada AM: "I play characters who live on the edge and I like that. I'm very aware that it's a very thin line between being inside jail and being outside jail."

Jeremy Irons, who won an Oscar, an Emmy, a Tony and a Golden Globe Award, became involved with Freeing the Human Spirit through the program's extraordinary octogenarian co-founder, Sister Elaine Macinnes, in the mid-nineties, during the time that Sr. Elaine was living in England. Irons took a Zen class that Sr. Elaine was teaching, and he was so inspired by her energy and dedication that he's been involved in prison service near his Oxford home for the past twelve years.

In 1993, Sr. Elaine was invited to Oxford to become Executive Director of the Prison Phoenix Trust, which sponsors meditation and Yoga classes in prison. A Catholic nun and Zen Master of the Sanbo Kyodan, based in Kamakura, Japan, Sr. Elaine spent thirty-two years in Asia learning the healing power and spiritual experiences that Yoga and meditation can bring to all, including prisoners. She began teaching meditation in prisons in 1980 while living in Manila, the Philippines, where she was asked by a group of political detainees in Bagong Bantay Detention Centre, who were being tortured, to teach them how to meditate. Observing how relaxed, energetic and sociable these angry, tense human beings became, Sr. Elaine became an fervent advocate of Restorative Justice and of prisons that would be true "correctional" facilities, places of help and healing, not only places of punishment. In 2003, she returned to Canada; and in 2004, she co-designed the FTHS program with Laurel Scott, a Yoga teacher and founding member of Yoga Outreach, which operates in southwestern British Columbia, teaching Yoga to men and women in correctional facilities.

Since its inception in 2004, Freeing the Human Spirit has established Yoga and meditation classes in fifteen Ontario prisons, and the staff is working hard to expand classes to as many facilities as possible. Classes are generally an hour and include a short introduction, gentle *Hatha Yoga* and thirty minutes of simple Zen meditation. FTHS offers four-week, eight-week and weekly programs, depending on the needs of the institution. Further prisoner support comes in the form of *Becoming Free*

through Meditation and Yoga, the program's 103-page manual.
Additionally, FTHS personnel correspond with individual
prisoners, encouraging them in their practices, and FTHS supplies
meditation mats and foam blocks to prisons and offers workshops
for its volunteer teachers, who are recruited through local Yoga
studios and meditation centers. What are its goals? According to
its website, FTHS's goals and objectives are:

- to promote and advance the physical, mental and spiritual
  development of prisoners in Canada through the practice of
  meditation and Yoga;

- to train, develop and support meditation and Yoga teachers who
  offer classes in correctional facilities;

- to develop and deliver a program of volunteer correspondents
  who will reply to letters from prisoners to support them in their
  practice.

FTHS states: "In each of our classes, we see evidence that
prisoners can change, discover their own inner self, become more
relaxed, discover ways to overcome their anger and frustration,
strengthen their self-discipline and become aware of a deepening
personal spirituality. This, in our view, is the very essence of
rehabilitation." The success of this program—the effectiveness of
both the practices and the volunteer instructors—is echoed in the
testimonies that appear on the website, testimonies like the one
from an inmate in a correctional facility called Maplehurst:

> Coming to the end of a not so short bit at Maplehurst, I feel the
> need this morning to thank all of those responsible for bringing
> the program here and a special heartfelt thanks to Glenn who,
> week after week and ever so humble, helps a few of us to find
> a tranquil refuge in a harsh and monotonous existence. Glenn
> has [been] and is a skilled guide into the basics of Yoga and
> Meditation. His insights and conversations, though brief, have
> been inspiring. I will leave here a little richer and, definitely,
> with a little more peace in my heart. Thank you!

As Jeremy Irons told his Canada AM interviewer: "When you're
banged up in prison . . . you're stuck in a cell on your own; a very

negative experience . . . . But if you can turn that cell into an *ashram*, if you can learn to meditate and do Yoga, exercise your mind and exercise your body, then it becomes a positive experience."

Prison Phoenix Trust

The Prison Phoenix Trust, founded by Ann Wetherall, has a small office in Oxford, England, which is staffed by two full-time and five part-time workers, along with twenty volunteers. Also, there are some ninety Yoga teachers countrywide who are offering weekly Yoga and meditation classes in prisons.

Having heard accounts of spiritual experiences among prisoners, Wetherall felt inspired to offer inmates the rich benefits of Yoga and meditation.

The Prison Phoenix Trust supports those who write in for help in their spiritual lives or in response to what they've heard about the Trust's work. Specially trained "letter-writers," mostly volunteers, answer some 2,000 letters a year from prisoners. They correspond with the prisoner for as long as he or she wishes, even after the prisoner is released from prison, and they offer prisoners support and encouragement to practice daily meditation in their cells. Another aspect of the Trust's service is to find and train qualified teachers to establish Yoga and meditation classes in prison. Classes are arranged in close collaboration with prison administrators and at least two prison governors attend classes; in fact, of the 134 weekly classes currently being held, twenty-five are for prison officers and staff.

In "A Precious Freedom," an article that appeared online in *Resurgence* (issue 235, 2006), writer Shirley Du Boulay, author of *The Cave of the Heart*, describes the inspiring work of the Prison Phoenix Trust. Du Boulay recounts the Trust's claim that a cell need not only be a place of incarceration and restriction, but that it can also be "a place where the spirit can find freedom, even joy." Apparently, John Graham agrees. A troubled adolescent, at age sixteen, Graham was sent to a school for delinquents, and from twenty-six to forty-five years old he was trapped in a pattern of drug addiction and incarceration. Ten years later, at fifty-five, he was a free man, and he says that the greatest thing that ever happened to him was his introduction to meditation, when "the stark nature of the prison suddenly became a sacred place."

How do prisoners get to know about the Trust? They usually find out through the prison grapevine or through the Trust's advertisement in the prison newspaper. It does take courage on the inmates' part to join the program and to meditate, because others might be quick to mock them. Normally, those who seek out the program feel that they've hit bottom and can't sink any lower; their past is bleak, their present is bleak and their future seems even bleaker. However, the Prison Phoenix Trust knows from experience that this state of mind, with all its pain and suffering, can be an opportunity for change and self-transformation. To illustrate this point, Du Boulay ends her piece with a quote from a prisoner who was serving a life sentence. Before he started meditating, he had been acting out aggressively, fighting with prison officers and smashing things, seeing life as "a series of disasters punctuated by the odd catastrophe." While he's not exactly sure what he's found, he perceives life quite differently now: "It's a hell of a lot more than I had in addiction. The lotus grows with its roots in mud and still produces a beautiful bloom. I finally get that!"

Reformation of Prisoners in India

Today, the benefits of Yoga are recognized and experienced everywhere, and Yoga is being taught in many prisons around the world to help prisoners manage stress and anger, stay healthy–mentally and physically–and transform negative thinking and habits. But what's happening in India, where Yoga originated? Do prisoners there have access to their own homegrown, holistic system of self-reformation, self-rehabilitation and, ultimately, self-transformation? Happily, the answer is a resounding yes!

Tamil Nadu, India

Tamil Nadu is a large state in South India–its capital is Chennai, formerly Madras–where concerted efforts are taken to improve the general welfare of prisoners. In fact, according to the Tamil Nadu Prison Department website, the government accords the utmost priority to the administration of prisons. Thus, the state's prison department is sanctioned to provide reformation and rehabilitation training for inmates through a program, apparently the first of its kind in the country, called Prisoners' Adalat.

Listing the training possibilities offered to prisoners, first on the website's list is "Yoga and Meditation," with the explanation that Yoga and meditation classes are conducted regularly "in order to transform the lives of prisoners." The classes are provided by about a dozen non-government organizations–to all inmates incarcerated in Tamil Nadu prisons.

Additional training includes academic education, from elementary through secondary school, as well as higher education correspondence courses that are conducted by various universities. Prisons also provide industrial and vocational training and NGOs make certified computer training courses available.

Bihar School of Yoga, Munger, Bihar, India

The Bihar School of Yoga was founded in 1964 by Paramahamsa Satyananda. According to the school's website, the Yoga techniques developed there synthesize many approaches to personal development and are based on traditional Vedantic (from the sacred Hindu writings of the Vedas), *tantric* (from *Tantra*, an esoteric Hindu tradition based on certain disciplines, rituals and meditation practices) and Yoga teachings combined with contemporary physical and mental health sciences.

In addition to the training offered at the Bihar Yoga Bharati, the Bihar School of Yoga guides Yoga projects and medical research in association with hospitals and organizations. Moreoever, its programs are being utilized in both the public and private sectors, as well as in the educational field and in prisons.

In the November 6, 1999 issue of *Yoga Magazine*, Sannyasi Janaki, wrote an informative article entitled "Benefits of Yoga for Prison Inmates," where she describes a pilot study initiated by Swami Niranjanananda Saraswati of the Bihar School of Yoga. The study was carried out in 1994 with the participation of a small group of prisoners incarcerated in the Munger District Jail. The purpose of the study was for prisoners to utilize Yoga practices to harmonize their bodies and minds so that they could effectively cope with stressful situations. Attendance at the daily classes was voluntary. After the fifteen-day program ended, the prisoners reported the following results: a general feeling of freshness and relief from chronic bowel problems and insomnia, reduced hostility, anxiety and frequency of negative emotions and a more positive attitude toward life, toward fellow prisoners and toward the authorities. The program was extended to three more jails, and the results reported in the pilot study were confirmed by the prisoners in these jails. Because of the program's success, the government of Bihar asked the Bihar School of Yoga to extend the program to other prisons, and by 1995, the program was taught in 24 jails to 1,013 prisoners, all of whom attended voluntarily.

Prisoners were given questionnaires before and after the Yoga training program. The questions dealt with physical, mental and emotional health, addiction, interpersonal interactions and future plans. The results indicated improvement in physical fitness, energy levels, strength, flexibility and better digestion and sleep; reduced feelings of anger, revenge, anxiety, depression and interpersonal conflict; increased feelings of happiness, peace and altruism; a more positive outlook on life; and a decreased desire for tobacco. Asked what they planned to do after their release from prison, over 63 percent of the inmates wanted to work and live a normal family life, 16 percent wanted to lead a spiritual life and work for social upliftment and 2.08 percent wanted to take revenge against enemies.

Sannyasi Janaki points out yet another benefit: the cost of prison medical expenditure was reduced.

In response to these encouraging results, the Home Department of the Government of Bihar decided to extend the training to all the jails in Bihar. Since a great number of trained Yoga teachers would be needed, officials decided to train prisoners who were serving life sentences to become Yoga teachers and to send them to different prisons throughout the state.

A one-month Teacher Training Course began in 1996 in all eight Bihar central jails (preference was given to volunteers who had previously taken the Yoga training). The 167 prisoners who passed the Yoga Teachers Test received a Yoga Instructors Certificate. And the results of their questionnaires indicated the following: 85 percent reported that they were more physically fit, mentally happier and more alert; 95 percent enjoyed better sleep and improved digestion; 70 percent had a substantial reduction, and 20 percent a slight reduction, in such negative emotions as anger, revenge, anxiety, depression; 85 percent reported an increase in altruistic and pro-social behavior; 83 percent cited a reduction in interpersonal conflicts; 98 percent resolved to continue their Yoga practices; and 95 percent expressed the desire to teach Yoga to fellow prisoners.

As Sannyasi Janaki states in her article, the reports obtained from each prison regarding perceived changes in health and behavior confirmed that Yoga had brought about positive changes in the physical and mental health and conduct of the prisoners. She also informs us that, unfortunately, this program came to a halt because of a change in government in Bihar and because of decreased interest in social welfare programs.

On the other hand, she cites other Indian prison success stories. In one prison, for example, a Yoga teacher taught two Yoga sessions daily for four weeks. At the end of the month, he asked the students for feedback. All reported increased self-confidence and the willingness to return to society to deal with the shame of their imprisonment. Apparently, some of them were innocent and had previously declared that they would rather die in prison than return home to face insults and accusations. Other students were gang members who said that they were helped by *Yoga Nidra* (deep relaxation, *Ajapa Japa* (repetition of a sacred sound) and *Mouna* (maintaining silence), all practices that enabled them to calm their mind and to differentiate between good and bad. Also, the superintendent and jail personnel noticed that the students were less aggressive, quieter and more positive.

In another prison, a particularly angry inmate threatened that once he was released, he would kill the person responsible for putting him in jail. The Yoga teacher insisted, "First do Yoga, then kill him!" He asked the man to do 25 rounds of *brahmari* (humming breath) in the morning and in the evening. Finally, at the end of the month-long program, when he was due to be released, instead of wanting to kill the person, this student wanted to stay in prison for another six months to practice Yoga. The superintendent agreed, provided the inmate taught Yoga to other prisoners. Eventually, the fellow wrote to his Yoga teacher, acknowledging that Yoga had brought him great happiness and satisfaction, because he was now able to help others.

Doing Time, Doing Vipassana

Currently, probably the most widely-known and successful prison reformation/rehabilitation programs in India is the ten-day Vipassana meditation course that evolved through the initiative and dedication of Kiran Bedi, a former Inspector General of prisons.

Apparently, Vipassana meditation was first tried in prison in the mid-1970s, with two ten-day courses conducted for officials and inmates of a prison in Jaipur, in the State of Rajasthan. Despite the success of these programs, no further courses were carried out in India for almost twenty years. But in 1993, the newly appointed Inspector General of Indian prisons, Kiran Bedi, during the process of reforming the harsh Indian penal system, learned about the Vipassana courses that had been conducted in the 70s, and she requested that courses be conducted in the largest prison in India, Tihar Jail, outside of New Delhi. The results were dramatic. And based upon the success of these courses, another course was conducted in 1994 by Mr. S. N. Goenka and several of his assistant teachers for over a thousand inmates of Tihar prison, with extraordinary results for all those who participated.

The prison documented the effects perceived by the prisoner-students at the completion of the course: 96 percent asserted that they were now able to control their anger, and 4 percent stated that the frequency of their anger had been reduced, although the intensity remained the same; 90 percent achieved peace of mind and no longer experienced stress for petty reasons and for reasons beyond their control; 96 percent learned to concentrate their mind on the subjects of their choice; 100 percent developed compassionate and benevolent feelings toward other inmates and staff members; 48 percent gave up smoking; 98 percent felt physically fit after the course; 66 percent stopped dwelling on the unpleasant past, concerning themselves more about the present; 70 percent started planning for a brighter future upon release; 86 percent gave up self-centeredness and started cooperating with and helping fellow inmates; and 100 percent stated that such programs should be organized periodically.

Kiran Bedi, the highest ranking woman in the Indian Police Service, is fearless, compassionate and innovative, admired and loved in India and internationally. Not only did this extraordinary trailblazer bring Vipassana meditation into the prisons, evoking much change and many initiatives, she also introduced a holistic approach to personal growth and reformation.

The Vipassana meditation program continues today and, thanks to the award-winning documentary about the program, *Doing Time, Doing Vipasana,* many people have become aware of the efficacy of such programs and have brought them into prisons in other countries.

Doing Time, Doing Vipassana was filmed during the winter of 1994 to 1995 by Israeli filmmakers Ayelet Menahemi and Eilona Ariel, who traveled to Tihar Jail and Baroda Jail in the State of Gujerat, where Vipassana courses had also been introduced. Menahemi and Eilona conducted and filmed extensive interviews with prison officials, including Kiran Bedi, and with inmates from many different countries who participated in the courses. They created a powerful and inspiring 52-minute documentary showing how Vipassana meditation has been successfully employed to change, dramatically, the attitude and behavior of the inmates and jailers who participated in the courses, improving the entire atmosphere of the prison environment. *Doing Time, Doing Vipassana* received the San Francisco International Film Festival's Golden Spire Award, the INTERCOM (International Communications Film & Video Competition, Chicago) Silver Plaque Award and the American National Council on Crime &

Delinquency (NCCD) Award for its contribution toward raising public awareness of the issue of prisoner reformation/rehabilitation and how this issue affects society in general.

Doing Time, Doing Vipassana is still widely distributed and showings are sometimes followed by a discussion led by local Vipassana meditators.

Isha Foundation

Located in Coimbatore, Tamil Nadu, India (the birthplace of Sri Gurudev Swami Satchidananda) and founded by Sadhguru Jaggi Vasudev, the Isha Foundation is a dynamic organization that sponsors Inner Freedom for the Imprisoned–a prison outreach Yoga program that focuses on inner transformation. Isha Foundation's Yoga prison programs help inmates develop emotional and mental balance, along with communication skills that they can use to improve the quality of their life during incarceration and to increase their chance for success when they return to the larger society.

After a pioneering program for life-term prisoners at the Coimbatore Central Prison, Isha Foundation Yoga programs were conducted in several other South Indian prisons at the request of the Inspector General of Prisons. These programs were also carried out in 2002, for the first time, in two American correctional facilities: the Pennsylvania Department of Corrections at Waymart and the Luther Luckett Correctional Complex in La Grange, Kentucky. According to the Isha Foundation website, prisoners experienced such an amazing transformation that some of the prison guards who were present wanted to participate in the programs. Indeed, the programs were so successful that both prisons requested that the programs be continued at their sites and Pennsylvania officials asked Sadhguru Jaggi Vasudev to expand the program to all twenty-seven Pennsylvania state prisons.

Art of Living Foundation

The July 19, 2007 issue of Business Daily Africa featured an article by Beatrice Gechenge entitled "Yoga: Part of Correction in Kenyan Prisons." The article focuses on a program administered and conducted by the Art of Living Foundation (AOLF) at Kamiti, Thika and Lang'ata Women's prisons in Kenya.

According to Gechenge, Chrisanthus Makokha, Chief Officer one at the Prison Headquarters, believes that Yoga is working well with the prison's rehabilitation program, as prisoners were enthusiastic about taking the meditation training. He also verified that discipline in the prisons had improved, prompting headquarters to install the AOLF program in all prisons in the country. Ms. Namratta Shah, an AOLF trainer in Kenya, reported that some twenty-five prisoners who had gone through the training were released for good conduct. Regarding the aim of the program, Ms. Shah stated, "We want to empower them to control their addictions and ensure that they don't drift to crime and, at the same time, be in a position to train other youths."

Another significant benefit of the program is that AOLF channels the proceeds from the cost of the program to training for the poor and to other prison programs.

You Can Always Be Happy and Healthy–Just Remold Your Life!

The prison programs included here represent a small sampling of Yoga and meditation programs designed to serve prisoners, to give them the tools that can help them experience true freedom, the inner freedom that comes through peace of mind. (For a comprehensive listing of Yoga teachers and organizations working with prisoners, as well as related books, articles and videos, see "Yoga in Prison" in the "Resources" section in the back of this book.) The time-honored teachings and practices of Yoga transform negative thinking into positive thinking, so that prisoners come to realize that their incarceration is an opportunity for spiritual growth and that their suffering is a means of purification, a burning out of the impurities of body and mind, a process of refinement on every level of being. A long time ago, the Indian sage Acharya Shankara taught that a human being's goal is to live in complete peace and joy as a liberated one. That "one" refers to each and every one of us, no matter on which side of the fence we may find ourselves during this lifetime.

Chapter 6
The Heart of the Matter

*We should feel that the whole world is ours. Wherever you feel it
is necessary to help, go there and work. This practice is needed today.
Through sharing and caring, we find ease within ourselves and among
our fellow beings.* —Sri Swami Satchidananda

Widening Our Circles of Compassion

In its Penal Reform Briefing No. 2, 2007, Penal Reform
International (PRI), a non-profit organization based in The
Netherlands, reports that, for many, imprisonment is marked by the
deterioration in health and well-being The report states that prison
populations characteristically represent the most disadvantaged and
marginalized sections of society, whose members generally have a
low health status. Moreover, PRI asserts that all prisoners have a
right to health, no matter what their legal status and that "the human
right to health is related to and dependent upon the realization of
other human rights, such as the right not to be tortured or ill-treated,
the right to recognition as a person before the law and to a fair trial,
the right to food and the right to education and training.

In this book, I have set out to illustrate that Yoga has proven
itself to be an effective method in training prisoners to rehabilitate
themselves on every level: the physical, the psychological, the
intellectual, the social and the spiritual. Obviously, it will take more
than Yoga to reform and transform our prison systems. But at least
we can start with our prison inmates, whose well-being, in no small
way, impacts the well-being of the larger society to which many of
them will return.

On the Insight Prison Project website, it says that more
than twenty years ago, when the State of California enacted
legislation stating that "the purpose of imprisonment for crime
is punishment" (Penal Code 1170 (a) (1), it essentially banned
rehabilitation from the state's penal system. Since that time,
according to IPP, the number of California's prisons has increased
by 554 percent, the average cost to house, feed and guard an
inmate in a state prison is almost $30,000 a year, and almost

70 percent of those who leave prison return within two years of release. And how do the state's citizens feel about this disquieting state of affairs? According to IPP, a recent survey conducted in California by the National Council on Crime and Delinquency "showed that the general public feels that the 'punishment only' system has failed and is strongly in favor of spending Correctional monies on rehabilitation."

The good news is that IPP, in collaboration with the San Quentin State Prison is working to bridge the gap between punishment and parole through a unique rehabilitation program that includes Yoga instruction. And since we're on the subject of prisoner rehabilitation in the State of California, this is a good time to recount the story of Jeri Becker, who served twenty-three years and four months in a California prison.

Jeri's Tale. Jeri's tale begins in March of 1980, when she went to a houseboat in Sausalito to pick up drugs that she had already paid for. She was accompanied by a male friend who had brought along a gun. The friend got into an argument with the drug dealer, the two fought for the gun, and the dealer was fatally wounded. According to trial testimony, the friend pointed the gun at the dealer's girlfriend, but Becker successfully pleaded for the woman's life. Strangely—at least to me—Jeri Becker's gun-toting friend was convicted of second-degree murder, while Becker was convicted of first-degree murder, receiving a 25-year-to-life prison sentence. As you can imagine, her life was transformed—in more ways than one: during her time in prison, Jeri Becker became a yogi. With respect to Jeri's transformation, the following letter, dated July 15, 1984 and addressed to Swami Satchidananda, speaks for itself.

Beloved Swamiji,

Namaste. I have been wanting to write to you for so very long but just never seemed to know how to start with words. I am incarcerated in a California state prison for women. I am serving my fourth year of a 25-year-to-life sentence for the crime of being aboard a boat when two men got into a fight and one was fatally wounded.

I have been interested in, and attracted to, Yoga ever since I first read of Paramahansa Yogananda over 20 years ago, though I never dedicated my life to any particular path. My real understanding of Yoga actually began during the year I spent in a jail cell in 1980. But of all the books, etc. which came my way to read and study, none so touched me personally as your biography. Here in prison, I continued to practice the *asanas*, meditate (I've learned to meditate amidst quite an array of noise, distractions and chaotic energies). The more I practice, the more practice I need. But the purpose of this letter is really to tell you a story about an experience I had about a year ago, which you may or may not be aware of.

On Christmas day, 1982, an administrative decision was made here to deem me a high security risk, because of my long sentence, and to place me in the "hole" (i.e., isolation) for an indefinite period. More "dancing lessons" from God! The "hole" here is just an empty cell where one always remains locked in and few personal articles are allowed. After a time, I managed to get a few inspirational books, including several back issues of *Integral Yoga Magazine*; and because I draw, I managed to get some paper and colored pencils. During this time, I wrote to the Integral Yoga Center closest to the prison, hoping that someone might be able to visit me from there (not realizing then that I was soon enough going to be able to be receptive and open enough to have a regular "visitor"). Anyway, in response to my letter, Rev. Pushpa Engle sent me some photographs of you, including one small 2-1/2 x 3 laminated photo of your face with a picture of the proposed LOTUS on the reverse side.

My time in the "hole" (which lasted ten months) became a great opportunity for the "full-time" spiritual practices that I felt so hungry for; it was nearly like being on retreat, albeit a bit noisy. I managed to get by on the debilitated food, slid through a slot in the door, by picking out any vegetables, rinsing them and repeating the *mantra* of the Buddha while chewing in order to re-vitalize them and by practicing extended periods in *Yoga Nidra*, concentrating especially on sending life-force throughout the body from my solar plexus. Sometimes (now this doesn't describe easily within the limitations of words), even the movement of a spider on the cell bars or a rivulet of rainwater glimpsed through the bars would be invested with the energy of your teaching, and there would be a clear lesson therein.

To sum this up, what I experienced during those months in isolation was a very real bond with your energy, teachings, etc. (Another aspect of your teachings, incidentally, which I *especially* enjoy is your marvelous "play" with English words!) One of the products of the creative energy passing through me in the "hole" was a portrait that I drew of you, lovingly and happily, with colored pencils. I had always intended that the finished portrait would be a gift to you. But I enjoyed the portrait's "company" in isolation. Then, in August of 1983 (one year ago), I was finally released back to the main prison population, and the portrait was exhibited in some prison art shows, where it had a ribbon placed on it! I'm no longer able to display your portrait or any other pictures in my cell here as recent regulations prevent us from having much property in our cells and from having anything on the walls. So, again, a marvelous opportunity to practice non-attachment presents itself. Also, it is the spirit and energy within the heart—not physical pictures or images—that are of any consequence. With the guru's image in mind, the inspiration is always there, which brings me to my present situation.

Over the past year that I've been back on the main prison yard, I, of course, do not have the time, space and opportunities for solitude that I had in the "hole." I realize that this is not justification for becoming slack in practice; yet, I often allow my mind to get so busy and distracted here. I often lose touch with that incredible peace and "closeness" that I felt while in isolation. I have been conducting a weekly class in *Hatha Yoga asanas* for the past year—the "teachers" of the class are two Integral Yoga posture tapes that we practice to as a class. Sometimes, the number of participants dwindles to two or three, but, always, we keep that space open with the energy. (Of late, we have had five or six regular participants in the class—quite a crowd here.)

I have, finally, sent your pencil portrait (along with its ribbon) to an acquaintance in San Francisco who has promised to send it on to you. I am making a vow today to set aside meditation time each morning, again, so that, hopefully, by quieting this restless mind once again, I may achieve that "inner-connection" once again.

One of my favorite rituals described in your writings was that of the cracking of the coconut on a birthday. May I ask you for your blessing on my birthday this November 28th? (I will be 35 years old.)

In Love and Light,
Jeri Becker

Jeri Becker's stirring letter reached Gurudev at the new Satchidananda Ashram-Yogaville community in Virginia. Probably a week or so after hearing from Becker, Gurudev replied:

> Beloved Self Jeri,
> Love and blessings.

Thank you for your loving letter, which I was pleased to receive and to note the benefit that you have felt from my humble service and the great teachings of the yogic science.

Your words touched my heart, especially because philosophy is easy to read and quote but difficult to put into daily life. You have proved the greatness of Yoga in your very life. You are a yogi and have shown how God uses various situations and people to test us and draw us closer.

I often speak about how, with the proper attitude, even being in prison can feel like being on a "retreat." You have shown that this is possible and I am sure that your sincerity will bring you great growth and progress on the spiritual path.

I was also pleased to note that you are conducting Yoga classes at the prison. This is wonderful and I am glad that God is using you as a good instrument to serve and help many souls who are seeking inner peace.

I hope you do not mind that I shared your letter with many of our members here. I wanted to show them that it is possible even under really difficult situations to put the Yoga practices and teachings into play. They were all really touched by your experiences and have rededicated themselves to striving even more toward the goal. A few of the members came forward and donated money to pay for some books and a subscription to the *Integral Yoga Magazine* to be sent to you.

Continue to have faith in God and trust that all is for your highest good. With this kind of faith and devotion, nothing will be able to disturb your peace. You can face any situation. Know that I will keep you in my thoughts and prayers, and I wish you all success in your sincere efforts to realize the peace and joy within, which is your own true nature.

May you continue to share that peace and joy, love and Light with one and all.

Ever Yours in the Lord and Light,
Swami Satchidananda

According to Rev. Prem Anjali, who served for many years as Gurudev's assistant, Jeri Becker and Gurudev corresponded for many years. She regularly sent him letters, as well as beautiful cards and poems that expressed her appreciation of the Yoga teachings. He always sent his newest book or booklet along with his replies. In addition, Gurudev would send her, in care of the prison library, sets of books, audio and video tapes of *satsangs* and Yoga classes. As she began teaching Yoga to other inmates, Jeri would ask Gurudev for advice on how to be a vegetarian on a diet that had limited vegetarian options and for other inspiring advice that she could share with the other inmates. Furthermore, Gurudev sent letters petitioning for her release to the Governor of California and to the President, and he asked others who could help to join in the letter-writing campaign. Prem Anjali recalls that Gurudev would always say that Jeri was the perfect example of someone transforming his or her prison life into an *ashram* life. In fact, during his talks he referred to her often, inspiring his many listeners with his description of Jeri's positive attitude toward her incarceration.

As for me, I first encountered Jeri Becker when I served as editor of *Integral Yoga Magazine*, which published her letters and other writings. I was thoroughly impressed not only by Becker's strength of mind, her sense of purpose and her faith, but also by her commitment to self-rehabilitation and her loving service in helping other inmates help themselves.

During her incarceration at the California Institution for Women, Becker's record remained spotless; she became a prison social worker, ran a 12-step program, served as a Yoga instructor, a lay minister, a choir director and a peer counselor. A true yogi committed to self-discipline, self-transformation and, selfless service, Jeri Becker transformed her own life and didn't stop there. With steadfast devotion, she shared her knowledge, experience and enthusiasm with other inmates, inspiring them to turn their lives around, too. A campaign to win her release ensued. In fact, an article in the *San Francisco Chronicle* ("Killer to be freed after 23 years, Governor declines to block her parole," December 23, 2003) reported that "Becker's release was almost unparalleled in its scope and diversity, a grassroots effort fueled by Internet technology and old-fashioned faith in the power of human redemption. One of many ardent supporters was E. Warren McGuire, the Superior Court judge in Marin County. It was Judge McGuire who had sent Becker to prison. Over the years, McGuire became convinced that Becker had reformed and he lobbied for her release. And in 2002, the California Board of Prison Terms granted her parole. But Jeri Becker's drama–and *karma*–continued. In October of that year, a month before his re-election, Gov. Gray Davis reversed the parole board's decision (according to the article in the *San Francisco Chronicle*, Davis routinely overturned parole board decisions). However, when Becker, again, applied for parole in July of 2003, the new governor, Gov. Arnold Schwarzenegger declined to block her parole. Jeri Becker had earned her freedom.

Evidently, Gov. Schwarzenegger, who reviews each parole case individually, takes a humane and compassionate stance, recognizing that people who are incarcerated can and do reform themselves when they are given the transformative tools that lead to a healthy, creative and productive life. But how does the general public feel about prisoner rehabilitation?

Barry Krisberg and Susan Marchionna shared some encouraging–not to say enlightening–information gathered from a poll of US voters. In their article, "Attitudes of US Voters toward Prisoner Rehabilitation and Reentry Policies," which appeared in the April 2006 issue of *Focus*, an online publication of the National Council on Crime and Delinquency, they report: "By almost an 8 to1 margin (87 percent to 11 percent), the US voting public is in favor of rehabilitative services for prisoners as opposed to a punishment-only system. Of those polled, 70 percent favored services both during incarceration and after release from prison." And why do people feel this way? Because they think–at least a third (31 percent) of them do–that "released prisoners are more likely than they were before their imprisonment to commit future crimes, while only one in seven (14 percent) think that released prisoners "are less likely to commit future crimes. A majority of those polled (52 percent) feel that released prisoners "have the same likelihood after release to commit future crimes." Apparently, that's why a large majority, 70 percent, prefers to see that state-funded rehabilitation services are available to prisoners both while they are in prison and after they've been released from prison.

Obviously, the citizens who participated in the poll are sensible. They recognize that the rehabilitation of our prisoners is essential to the security and creative evolution of our society. One would also hope that these individuals are sensitive human beings, that they are aware of the reality expressed in a simple yet profound verse that I came across in a web publication called "The Voice of the Imprisoned" (www.prisoners.com):

> Prisoners
>> There are good people.
>> There are bad people.
>> They are, however,
>>> The same people.

Yes. Good or bad, we are all the *same* people. I italicized the word "same" to bring out the subtle allusion in this simple verse to the profound teaching that we are all, literally, the same; we are all human beings, and, on the most subtle level of being, we are all part and parcel of the same cosmic consciousness. Religions communicate this fact when they tell us that we are made in the image of God. Modern science is saying the same thing, using a different metaphor when it tells us that we–and everything else–are made of the same mysterious energy that permeates the universe. Yoga masters often illuminate this concept with the analogy that just as waves are individual expressions of the one ocean, all of us are individual expressions of the supreme consciousness. What this analogy is meant to convey is that, ultimately, we are all one; on the level of everyday life, the analogy illustrates that we are all interrelated, interdependent. And this is the heart of the matter, whether the issue is the exploitation of workers or global warming or universal healthcare or the depletion of natural resources or prisoner–and prison–reform. Our very survival and the survival of our planet depends on the realization that we are our brothers' and sisters' keepers, that is to say, that to be human is to care for one another, in every sense of the word. Caring for someone might mean removing people from the larger society and incarcerating them in prison. But caring for someone also means that we do whatever we have to do in the spirit of compassion. We care about them. If we have to punish someone, we do it because that person needs correction; we don't do it out of anger. We act, but our actions are grounded in empathy. When compassion and forgiveness inform our actions, even the worst characters can be transformed and sinners can turn into saints. Swami Satchidananda's spiritual master, Sri Swami Sivananda Maharaj, proved it.

Govindan's tale. Govindan was a young man who was permitted by Swami Sivananda to stay at the *ashram* for several months. On the evening of January 8, 1950, during the spiritual gathering, or *satsang*, Govindan approached the *satsang* hall from a dark entranceway and walked toward Swamiji with an axe in hand. He raised the axe, but as it came down, it struck the door. Govindan raised the axe, again, but this time the blade struck a picture that was hanging on the wall and only the handle struck Swamiji's turban. Normally, as soon as he entered the hall, Swamiji would remove the turban, but, that evening, he forgot. Thinking that what hit him was just a stick, he raised his hand, scratching it on the axe.

One of the swamis jumped up and grabbed Govindan, hugging him tightly so that he couldn't lift his hand again and he drew Govindan outside. The crowd in the hall immediately realized what had happened. Two people held Govindan while his hands and feet were bound. Then, some others started to beat him, but Swamiji shouted at the top of his voice: "Don't beat him, don't beat him." Govindan was taken to a nearby room and was locked in.

Swamiji instructed people to continue the chanting that was going on before the incident. Meanwhile, one of the swamis who had been in the hall had informed the other swamis, who ran to the police station and returned to the hall with a couple of policeman. Everyone went to the room where Govindan was being held. The rope that bound his hands and feet was removed. Swamiji went right up to Govindan and bowed to him with folded palms. He said, "Govindan, do you want to deal some more blows? Here I am. Kindly satisfy yourself." As the police inspector gazed at the scene in wonder, Govindan muttered, "No, I do not want to beat you any more. I am satisfied." As those assembled struggled to control their anger, Swami inquired, in a loving manner, "What harm did I do to you? Why did you get so angry with me? Govindan didn't reply.

Swamiji left and, with everyone following him, returned to his cottage. The police inspector asked whether he should lodge a complaint against Govinda, but Swami said no, that sending him away would be enough punishment. By this time, it was quite late, but people in the area had heard about the incident and many came rushing into the cottage with tears in their eyes. Swamiji received them as though nothing had happened; in fact, he was smiling radiantly.

The next day, it was decided that Govindan should be provided with train tickets to his native city. Before Govindan left, Swamji went to the police station with fruits, books, clothes, a new blanket and a *japa-mala* (prayer beads to use with *mantra* repetition) and he even prostrated before Govinda. Swamiji would not allow any suggestion that Govindan be charged with a crime, saying: "... No, I will not let the police charge Govindan. We should thank him for working out my *karma* so easily. The Lord has spared my life because there is some more service to be performed through this body. I must go on with that service. That is all the incident indicates to me."

A few weeks later, Swamiji received a letter from Govindan. Govindan wrote that he was grateful to Swamiji for what he had done, that he was praying that any other pitfalls that he might encounter be removed by Swamiji's grace and that he regarded himself as Swamiji's disciple. Swamiji smiled and said, "Put Govindan's name on the Magazine Free List ... All free literature should be sent to him. I will send him books; also, I will write to him to come again."

Through the years, Swami Sivananda encountered other angry, violent people. He always blessed and prayed that they would develop knowledge and inner spiritual strength. Eventually, they all returned to the *ashram* with a thorough change of heart, and he welcomed them with great love and affection. As Swamiji himself said, "It is not through compulsion or rules or regulations that men [and women] can be transformed into divine beings. They all must have convincing experiences of their own." To him, there was no person on this earth—even those considered to be the most evil—who didn't have his or her own good points. To him, no one was incorrigible. When he encountered those who were enslaved by bad habits, he encouraged them to practice *pratipaksha bhavana*, the yogic practice that emphasizes introducing good habits into one's life that will, eventually, push out the bad habits, the way we get rid of an automobile's old, dirty grease by simply pushing it out with new, clean grease. Through the transmission of his own dynamic spirit of sacrifice and unconditional love, Swami Sivananda inspired transformation in even the most downtrodden of human beings.

Throughout the ages and across the world, great spiritual beings have inspired and encouraged us to renounce the selfish desires and actions that prevent us from perceiving the unity of being and what Yogananda Paramahansa refers to as the "light of inner wisdom-guidance," which leads the way to true happiness. In fact, the brilliant Yoga master, Indian nationalist, poet, philosopher and spiritual guru, Sri Aurubindo, attained this realization of the One Self that permeates all creation while incarcerated in Alipore Jail. Sri Aurobindo, deeply involved in India's independence movement, was arrested in 1908 by British authorities on the suspicion that he was involved in a bomb threat, an allegation of which he was acquitted. It was in Alipore Jail that Sri Aurobindo had a profound spiritual experience, becoming aware of a "divine inner guidance."

Sri Aurobindo embraced the ancient science of Yoga, but his approach was a new one. Whereas yogis in the past retreated from the world, Sri Aurobindo remained in the world, maintaining that it wasn't necessary to withdraw from worldly life in order to experience self-realization. He called his new approach "Integral Yoga." And the central principle of his Integral Yoga is the evolution of consciousness. Sri Aurobindo taught that the aim of Yoga is the development of the inner self. This process, leading to the discovery of the One Self (Cosmic Consciousness) in all, will, ultimately, transform and divinize human nature. Sri Aurobindo expressed his expanded awareness and experience of the One Self in all in a most beautiful poem, composed in 1938, entitled "Cosmic Consciousness":

> I have wrapped the wide world in my wider self
> And Time and Space my spirit's seeing are.
> I am the god and demon, ghost and elf,
> I am the wind's speed and the blazing star.
>
> All Nature is the nursling of my care,
> I am its struggle and the eternal rest;
> The world's joy thrilling runs through me; I bear
> The sorrow of millions in my lonely breast.
>
> I have learned a close identity with all,
> Yet am by nothing bound that I become;
> Carrying in me the universe's call
> I mount to my imperishable home.

The reality that every human being–saint or sinner–is an integral part of the entire tapestry of life is echoed in the elegant prose of another brilliant and acclaimed twentieth-century figure, Dr. Albert Einstein:

"A human being is part of a whole, called by us the 'Universe,' a part limited in time and space. He experiences himself, his thoughts and feelings, as something separated from the rest–a kind of optical delusion of his consciousness. This delusion is a kind of prison for us, restricting us to our personal desires and to affection for a few persons nearest us. Our task must be to free ourselves from this prison by widening our circles of compassion to embrace all living creatures and the whole of nature in its beauty."
–*Albert Einstein*

How fortunate we are that in this new age of adversities and blessings, there are now hundreds, if not thousands of dedicated yogis on every continent who embrace the vision of such enlightened beings as those mentioned in this book and who care enough to impart the life-transforming teachings and practices of Yoga not just to those who have the freedom to travel to a class or to a weekend workshop, but also to those who are incarcerated in our many jails and prisons. As we can all imagine, prison life is intense, whether you're an inmate, a staff member, or a volunteer. And, as you've probably gathered, teaching Yoga and practicing Yoga in prison can be a formidable task. So, it might be helpful to remember that, sometimes, a little levity goes a long way. For example, when you teach or practice *pranayama*, the breathing practices, you might evoke the wisdom of an erudite Jewish Buddhist teacher:

Breathe in. Breathe out. Breathe in. Breathe out. If you forget to do this, attaining enlightenment will be the least of your problems.

Chapter 7
Converting Prison Life into *Ashram* Life

When I am self-contained and self-sufficient, there is nothing in the universe to interfere with my freedom. –Buddha

To those readers who are currently incarcerated: I hope that by now you've been assured that if you have the desire to live in permanent peace and joy, with a strong commitment to self-growth and a little imagination, you can make use of Yoga to free yourself from the shackles of an unrestrained mind. Then, as others have done before you and as many are doing today, you will, without a doubt, transform your prison experience into an *ashram* experience. If you're thinking: "Okay, I'm up for it, but where do I begin?" I'll give you a jump start.

Close your eyes, take a few deep inhalations and exhalations and relax. Then, introduce the thought that you will transform your prison into an *ashram*. Experience the power of your will, the force of your capability and the strength of your commitment to lead a healthy, happy, peaceful and productive life. Continue for five or ten minutes, and then open your eyes. Now, take a look at an ashram schedule and see how you can follow it–with any necessary adjustments, of course–right in prison. After the schedule, you'll find the format of our basic Integral Yoga Hatha Yoga class, along with some tips on meditation, *pranayama*, the yogic diet and the practice of keeping a spiritual diary.

Ashram Schedule

4:45 am	Wake up
5:00 am	*Pranayama*: Chant *OM* three times silently and then: 10 minutes of *kappalabati* (forceful diaphragmatic breathing) and 10 minutes of *nadi suddhi* (alternate nostril breathing).
	Meditation (½ hour)
5:45 am	*Hatha Yoga* (a classic session–including chanting, postures, deep relaxation and pranayama–lasts for 1 hour 20 minutes to 1 ½ hours)

8:00 am	Breakfast
8:30 am	Service
Noon	Meditation (½ hour)
12:45 pm	Lunch
1:45 pm	Service
5:00 pm	Optional *Hatha Yoga* session
6:00 pm	Meditation (15 minutes of *pranayama*, including *kappalaba*ti and *nadhi suddi*,with *nadhi suddi* leading into silent meditation)
6:30 pm	Supper
7:30 pm	Weekdays: scripture class twice a week; freetime Saturday night: *satsang* (spiritual gathering: lectures, concerts, performances, spiritual videos, discussions)
10: 00 pm	Bedtime

Hatha Yoga

Americans love change, invention and productivity, and, in their "new world," they thrive on adopting, and then transforming, "old world" traditions. This proclivity to "Americanize" foreign institutions is most salient in the area of food. Who else would come up with pineapple pizza, the croissantwich and the banana chocolate latte? So, it's no surprise that in the United States, where the once esoteric ancient Indian science of Yoga has pretty much become a mainstream pursuit and all too often thought of simply as a physical fitness activity, the traditional *Hatha Yoga* class has undergone various permutations that appeal to the ever-growing number of avid students. Nowadays, for example, one can find *Hatha* classes that integrate martial arts, dance and massage. A veritable *Hatha Yoga* smorgasbord.

Although Gurudev modified the classical Indian *Hatha Yoga* session to render it more suitable to Westerners–for instance, most of us aren't used to sitting cross-legged on the floor for long periods of time, so students are invited to adjust their posture when they need to; also, the Sanskrit chants that are done during the class include their English translations–Integral Yoga *Hatha* is based more on the classic model as it was practiced in India. At the same time, there's room for flexibility (pardon the pun) with regard to including poses, chants, or other practices that are not included in the standard Integral Yoga class, especially in the more advanced classes. Gurudev, who was himself a renowned *Hatha Yoga* master, or *Yogiraj*, offered this rule of thumb: any practice could be considered acceptable so long as that practice was not, *in any way*, harmful.

Another point that he emphasized was that while Yoga *asanas*, or postures, promote good health, they are not exercise. There is no strain, there is no pushing involved when doing *asanas*. In fact, *asana* simply means "posture," and in the *Yoga Sutras*, Sri Patanjali defines *asana* as "a steady, comfortable pose." Drawing on this definition, as well as years of study and practice, Gurudev taught that "Yoga *asanas* should be practiced with the utmost ease and comfort." The philosophy—and the wisdom—that underlies this teaching is that while we all come to the practices with our own capacity and may not, in the beginning, do them perfectly, regular practice will gradually lead to perfection. Practically speaking, when you don't hurry and you don't strain in a posture, you eliminate the risk of injury; and, at the same time, you're learning to discipline the mind.

In *Integral Yoga Hatha*, a classic (it was first published in 1970), comprehensive book of Hatha Yoga poses and practices, you can find photos of Gurudev demonstrating the classic postures. Additionally, the benefits and recommended time limits for each *asana* are included. And Gurudev offers guidance to help students avoid injuries, along with some helpful hints on how best to approach and prepare for a *Hatha Yoga* session. Take a look at some of his most important guidelines:

Hatha Yoga can be done at any time during the day or evening. While it's particularly conducive when done in the morning, when the stomach is almost empty, beginners will probably find their bodies more flexible in the evenings.

Hatha Yoga should always be practiced at least 2 ½ hours after a light meal.

When it comes to what to wear, nowadays, there's a whole line of fashionable clothing for *Hatha Yoga*. But, really, any comfortable, non-restricting pants or shorts and tops will work; in other words, you wouldn't want to do *Hatha* in a pair of stiff jeans with a tight belt around the waist.

During the *asana* practice, the breath should not be retained for a long time. Sometimes, the breath may stop for a moment, for example while raising your legs in the Plough pose (*Halasana*) or in Shoulder Stand (*Sarvangasana*) or in the Forward Bend (*Paschimothanasana*), and that's fine. Also, during the stomach lift (*Uddhiyana Bandha*) and during the Isolation and Rolling of the Abdominal Recti (*Nauli Kriya*), retention of the breath occurs quite naturally.

In general, while doing the *asanas*, it's good to exhale as you bend forward and to inhale as you bend backwards, breathing normally at all other times. And it's better to breathe through the nose and not the mouth, except when doing *Sitali* (Cooling Breath) and *Sitkari* (Wheezing Breath), at which times you would inhale through the mouth. It helps to remember that the nose is for breathing and the mouth is for eating and talking.

The basic Integral Yoga *Hatha* class for beginners opens with chanting; the class chants the syllable *OM* three times together to balance the mind and to create a feeling of unity. Then, the instructor leads responsive chanting of *Hari OM*, a *mantra*, or sound vibration that stimulates the body's energy. The class flows in the following sequence:

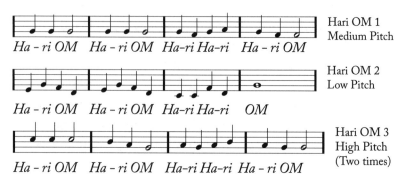

Netra Vyāyamam: Eye Movements

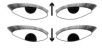 **Vertical:** Sit in a cross-legged position with the spine erect and head still. Move the eyes up and then down as far as possible without strain. Repeat a few times; then close and relax the eyes.

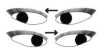 **Horizontal:** Move the eyes horizontally straight across the center of the vision from far right to far left. Repeat a few times, then close and relax the eyes.

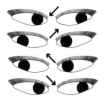 **Diagonal:** Move the eyes from the upper right to the lower left corner of the vision a few times, then repeat from upper left to lower right. Close and relax the eyes.

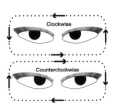 **Full Circle:** Move the eyes clockwise in a full circle, passing through all points on the circle. Repeat 3–4 times, then close and relax the eyes. Reverse, moving eyes counterclockwise, 3–4 times.

Now with eyes closed, rub the palms briskly together until they are very warm. Cup them over the eyes, blocking out all light. Feel the darkness and let your eyes absorb the warmth. When they feel fully relaxed, bring the fingertips to the eyes and lightly stroke the eyelids outward toward the ears a few times. Return the hands to the lap, and feel the effects.

Benefits: Exercises and relaxes eye muscles, increases circulation, tones the optic nerves and is a general aid to the improvement of the eyesight. Prepares the brain for experiential learning and can reduce depression.

Sūrya Namaskāram: Sun Salutation

Sometimes referred to as the Sun Worship–it derives from an ancient Indian temple dance–*Sūrya Namaskara* is made up of twelve positions, each one flowing into the next; Generally, at least in a Beginners class, the instructor leads the class through three rounds, but you can always add more rounds.

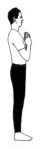

#1: Place the feet parallel, either together or a comfortable distance apart, palms together in front of the chest. Exhale.

#2: Inhale. Lock the thumbs, stretch the arms out and up alongside the ears. Stretch up and gently bend back from just below the shoulder blades.

#3: Exhale. Hinge forward from the hips, keeping the back flat, arms alongside the ears, knees soft. Lengthen the spine, and relax the head and arms toward the floor.

#4: Inhale. Bend the knees and place the hands on the floor outside the feet. Stretch the left leg far back, left knee on the floor. Release the pelvis down, move the chest forward, elongate the spine and look forward.

#5: Exhale. Bring the right foot back even with the left, buttocks raised high, flattening the back so the body forms an inverted "V" shape. Relax the crown of the head toward the floor. Draw the hips away from the hands, lengthen the spine and lower the heels toward the floor.

#6: Inhale. Lower the knees, leaving the pelvis slightly raised. Place the chest and chin on the floor with the hands beneath the shoulders.

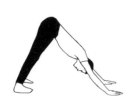

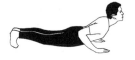

#7: Retain the breath. Shift the body weight forward, lowering the pelvis and abdomen to the floor. Elongate the spine and stretch up the head, neck and chest without pressing on the palms.

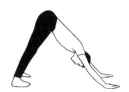

#8: Exhale. Press into the hands, and raise the buttocks again to form an inverted "V." Lengthen the spine and relax the heels toward the floor.

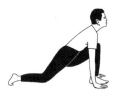

#9: Inhale. Swing the left foot forward between the hands, right knee to the floor. The front knee is above the ankle. Release the pelvis downward, move the chest forward, elongate the spine and look forward.

#10: Exhale. Bring the right foot forward even with the left. Straighten the knees if comfortable. Lengthen the spine and relax the head toward the floor.

#11: Inhale. Lock the thumbs, stretch the arms out alongside the ears and, bending the knees if necessary, flatten the back and stretch outward and upward. Bend slightly backward from just below the shoulder blades while looking at the hands.

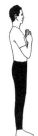

#12: Exhale. Stand erect, and bring the palms together at the chest. Lower the arms, step the feet apart, and relax.

Time: Begin with 3 rounds; gradually increase to as many as 12 according to your capacity. Do not overexert; stop before perspiring.

Benefits: A general tonic for entire body and personality, as it is a complete combination of bodily postures, breathing and prayerful attitude. Performed rapidly, it makes you alert; done slowly, it quiets the restless body and mind.

Some Optional Standing Poses

1. *Trikoṇāsana:* Triangle Pose

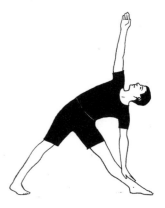

Take a comfortably wide stance. Turn the left foot out about 90 degrees and the right foot slightly inward while maintaining comfort, especially in the right knee. Place the palms on the hips and turn the torso forward while keeping the left knee in line with the left foot, allowing the right hip to move forward slightly if necessary. Inhale again to lengthen the spine and bring the arms to shoulders level. Exhale, hinge from the hips, leaning toward the left. Keep the back leg engaged, with the outside of the back foot in contact with the floor as the left arm is lowered to the shin, and raise the right arm overhead. Look at the upraised arm if comfortable; otherwise, look toward the left foot.

To exit the pose, on an inhalation while leading with the raised arm, raise the torso up, and bring the arms back to shoulder level. Release the arms to the side, and face both feet forward and relax.

Reverse foot positions and repeat on the right side.

2. *Naṭarājāsana:* King Dancer Pose

Stand erect. Shift the weight to the left foot. Bend the right knee and lift the right foot to take hold of the ankle or foot behind you with the right hand. Press the right foot back into the hand, drawing the thigh back and up. Keep both hips pointing forward. Raise the left arm toward the ceiling alongside the ear.

To exit, lower the arm, then the leg, and gently release the foot.

Repeat on the other side.

Śavāsana: Corpse Pose

The Corpse Pose, or *śavāsana*, is also known as the relaxation pose and is done in between the asanas. It's sometimes said that *śavāsana* is the most difficult of all the asanas, especially in our fast-paced modern society, because people–even children–find it difficult to let go and relax completely.

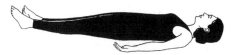

Technique: Lie on the back with the feet about shoulder width apart and the arms slightly away from the body with the palms facing upward. Close the eyes.

Mentally go through the body from the feet to the head, or the head to the feet. If you find any tension, mentally send a message to that part of the body to relax completely. Let the breath be relaxed.

Time: Allow quiet time of at least 30 seconds for relaxation.

Benefits: Allows all the muscles to relax and the energy to flow freely. Gives the body a chance to totally relax between poses.

Adhvāsana: Prone Pose

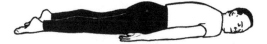

Technique: Roll over onto the abdomen. Turn the cheek to the side, arms alongside the body with the palms up, feet a comfortable distance apart, and relax.

Time: Allow quiet time of at least 30 seconds for relaxation.

Benefits: Same as the Corpse Pose, with the addition of helping to relieve soreness and muscle tightness in the neck.

Bhujaṅgāsana: Cobra Pose

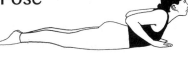

Technique: Lying facedown, bring the forehead to the floor.

Place the palms on the floor under the shoulders, elbows raised and close to the trunk, legs together and toes pointed. On the next inhalation, extend the head forward by lengthening the back of the neck, and without pressing into the hands, slowly raise the head, neck and chest, gradually raising the chest and arching the back. Keep the pelvis on the floor and come up only as far as the back can support the weight without pain.

To release, on an exhalation, roll down slowly, one vertebra at a time. Lower the chin and bring the forehead to the floor. Turn the cheek to the side and relax with the feet apart.

Time: 2 times, holding 15 seconds each time or once holding 30 seconds. Gradually lengthen to once for one minute.

Benefits: Develops flexibility in the chest. Strengthens the deep and superficial muscles of the back and neck. Increases abdominal pressure, thereby toning the abdominal organs and relieving sluggishness of the bowels. Pulls every vertebra and its attached ligaments backward and gives them a fresh supply of blood. Makes minor adjustments of the vertebrae. Releases nervous energy up and down the spinal column. Relieves back fatigue. Stretches abdominal muscles. Tones reproductive organs. Improves the posture and stretches the lungs.

Ardha Śalabhāsana: Half Locust Pose

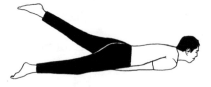

Technique: Lying facedown, bring the chin to the floor. Tuck the arms underneath the body, elbows close together and palms facing the thighs, floor or in gentle fists. Stretch the right leg out. Inhale and slowly raise the leg while keeping the weight centered on both hips. Keep the knee straight. Lengthen the lower back while extending out the leg and through the foot. On the next exhalation, continue to lengthen and slowly lower down the leg. Repeat with the left leg, and then repeat both.

Time: Twice with each leg, holding 10–15 seconds each time. This is a preparation for the following pose.

Śalabhāsana: Full Locust Pose

Technique: As above but steady the body and raise both legs. Keep the knees straight.

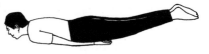

Time: Once, 15 seconds, gradually increasing the length of the hold.

Benefits: Tones the sympathetic nervous system and the liver. Develops strength in the lower back. Tones the areas of the lower back, pelvis and abdomen. The vertebrae of the lumbo-sacral region get a rich supply of blood. Intra-abdominal pressure is very high, toning the viscera and relieving constipation. Full pulmonic pressure forces open idle cells of the lungs, promoting elasticity of the lungs.

Dhanurāsana: Bow Pose

Contraindication: Not to be practiced by those with stomach or intestinal ulcers, high blood pressure or hernia.

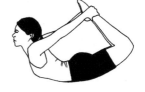

Technique: Lying facedown, bring the forehead to the floor. Bend the knees and take hold of the ankles. Have the knees and feet apart and parallel if possible. If comfortable in this preparatory position, keep the arms straight, and on the next inhalation, press the feet into the hands lifting the lower half of the body. Then slowly raise the head, neck and chest, arching the back to allow the entire weight to fall on the abdomen. Keep the arms straight. To release, on an exhalation, slowly lower down. Resume *advāsana.* Then roll onto the back and take *śavāsana.*

Time: Once, 15–30 seconds, gradually working up to holding once for one minute.

Benefits: Gives all the benefits of Cobra and Locust plus reduces abdominal fat. The weight on the abdominal aorta sends a flush of blood to the abdominal organs. Relieves congestion of blood in the viscera, energizes digestion, relieves gastrointestinal disorders such as constipation and gas. Stretches pectoral muscles of the chest.

Jānuśīrshāsana: Head-to-Knee Pose

Technique: Lying on the back, stretch the arms overhead, lock the thumbs and sit up with as much control as possible. Lower the arms. Sit on the front of the sitting bones. Bending the left leg, place the sole of the left foot against the upper right thigh, heel pressing the perineum or against the inside of the right leg, which is still outstretched. On an inhalation, stretch the arms up, lengthen the spine and lock the thumbs. On an exhalation, slowly hinge forward from the hips, keeping the back as flat and extended as comfortable. When the lower back begins to round, release the arms taking hold of the extended leg or foot without straining the lower back. Relax the shoulders, neck and head.

To come up, lock thumbs, stretch out and raise up while lengthening without straining the lower back. Repeat over the opposite leg. Then roll back down to the floor into *savāsana*.

Time: Once over each leg, 30–60 seconds each.

Benefits: Helps to control sexual energy and to evacuate the bowels when held for a short time. (Holding the pose for a longer time may increase constipation.) Stretches the hamstrings and the lumbosacral region of the spine.

Paśchimottānāsana: Forward Bending Pose

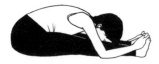

Contraindications: Not to be practiced if you have diseases of the abdominal viscera or an enlarged spleen.

Technique: Lying on the back with the arms stretched overhead, lock the thumbs and sit up with as much control as possible. Lower the arms. Sit on the front of the sitting bones with both legs outstretched. On an inhalation, stretch the arms up and lengthen the spine. On an exhalation, slowly hinge forward from the hips, keeping the back as flat and extended as comfortable. When the lower back begins to round, release the arms taking hold of the legs or feet without straining the lower back. Relax the shoulders, neck and head, and do not bounce or strain.

To come up, lock thumbs, stretch out and raise up while lengthening without straining the lower back. Then roll down to the floor and onto the back in *śavāsana*.

Time: Once, holding 60–90 seconds.

Benefits: Stretches nearly all posterior muscles. Tones the abdominal viscera. Helps cure hemorrhoids, constipation (if done for a short time), diabetes and prevents menstrual disorders. Stretches the thoracic spine and intercostal muscles of the ribs are stretched.

Sarvāṅgāsana: Shoulder Stand

Contraindications: Head, neck, shoulder and back injuries. Menses. Uncontrolled high blood pressure. Glaucoma. Recent surgery. Hiatal hernia. Presence of headache or fever.

Technique: Make sure there is no long hair or jewelry behind the neck, and tuck in your shirt. Please remember that you should not cough, sneeze or clear the throat while in the pose, or turn the neck from side to side. Lie on the back, arms alongside the body, palms down. With knees straight raise the legs to a 90-degree angle. Press on the palms, swing the legs slightly overhead and bring the hands immediately to support the back. Walk the elbows toward one another. Slowly bring the legs to the vertical position, bringing the chest as close as comfortable to the chin.

To lower out of the pose, slowly bring the straight legs over the head (bend the knees if desired), lower hands to the floor and slowly roll down the spine and then the legs with knees straight (or bent if desired).

Time: Once, 1–3 minutes.

Benefits: Pressure on the throat tones and massages the thyroid gland. Keeps the spine elastic, especially the cervical spine. Rests the legs and digestive organs. Improves venous blood flow, allowing the heart to work more efficiently. Allows abdominal organs to relax when back into their normal position. Improves circulation, nourishing spinal column and spinal nerves. Maintains healthy functioning of the reproductive, circulatory, digestive and respiratory systems. Coming into and out of the pose strengthens the abdominal muscles; holding the pose massages shoulder muscles and strengthens muscles of the lower back.

Matsyāsana: Fish Pose

Contraindications:
Not to be practiced if experiencing a headache or fever.

Technique: Lying on the back with the legs together, take hold of the sides of the thighs. Place the weight on the elbows. Without moving the elbows, sit up halfway and look down at the feet. Tilt the pelvis forward, giving the lower back a good arch. Inhale and expand the chest fully, arching the upper spine. Exhale and lower the crown of the head to the floor.

To come down put the weight on the elbows again, lift the head and back and lower slowly to the floor.

Time: Once, 20–60 seconds each (one-third of the time spent in *sarvāṅgāsana*).

Benefits: The thyroid and parathyroids in the throat area are massaged and toned. Apex of the lungs receives oxygen. Endocrine glands in the head (pineal and pituitary) are toned by the inversion of the upper body. The chest is greatly expanded aiding correct posture and respiration. This pose naturally massages congested parts of the neck and shoulders. The larynx and trachea are wide open. The upper spinal nerves are nourished. Coming into and out of the pose greatly strengthens the muscles of the neck, stretches the intercostal muscles of the ribs and builds the strength and elasticity of the lungs. This pose helps relieve hunchback, rounded shoulders and other posture problems.

Ardha Matsyendrāsana: Half Spinal Twist

Technique: Come to the front of the sitting bones. Draw the toes upward. Bend the right leg toward the chest. Cross the foot over the extended leg, placing the sole of the foot on the floor close to the knee. Bring the right arm behind the back and place the hand on the floor and centered. Wrap the front arm around the upraised knee, bringing the palm on or near the thigh. Or if you can keep the spine erect, bring the arm on the outside of the upraised thigh, and take hold of the extended leg. Grounding through both sitting bones, inhale and lengthen, exhale and initiate the twist at the level of the navel. Feel the twist move gradually up the spine; the head turning last. Slowly unwind and reverse the pose.

Time: Once on each side, 30 seconds or longer.

Benefits: Helps correct enlarged or congested liver or spleen, inactive kidneys and adrenals. Helps relieve dyspepsia, constipation, jaundice and obesity. Gives a vigorous twist to the spinal column, increasing flexibility along the entire spine. Gives the neck tendons a good twist. Each vertebra and its attached ligament get a fresh supply of blood. Contracts and tones the abdominal organs. Relieves pain or stiffness in the hip joints. Stretches the muscles of the buttocks. Excellent tonic for the sympathetic nervous system and nerves rooted in the spine.

Some Additional Optional Poses

1. *Pūrva Nāvāsana*: Boat Pose

Lie on the stomach, with the arms stretched overhead. Lock the thumbs if comfortable, and with head between the arms, raise both halves of the body, resting on the abdomen. To exit, lower down and take *adhvāsana*.

2. *Pavanamuktāsana*: Wind-Relieving Pose

Lie on the back. Bend the right knee and press it to the chest. Bring the face to the knee while retaining breath. Release and repeat with the left leg. Release and repeat with both legs.

3. *Jaṭhara Parivartanāsana*: Abdominal Twist

Lie on your back and bend the knees with the soles of the feet on the floor. Extend your arms out at shoulder level. Raise the hips slightly, move the hips a few inches to the right and return them to the floor. Inhale and bring the knees into the chest. Exhale and roll both legs to the left toward the floor. If comfortable, keep the right shoulder on the floor. Lift your head and turn it to the right. (If the rotation of the neck is uncomfortable, leave the head in the center.)

To exit, turn the head back to center, raise both legs back to the chest, and return the soles of the feet to the floor.

Repeat on the other side.

4. *Bhadrāsana*: Gentle Pose

Sit in a comfortable position with the spine erect. Bring the soles of the feet together allowing the knees to move downward toward the floor. Lace the fingers around the toes or ankles and gently press down on the inner thighs. With practice, rest the elbows on the inner thighs and bend forward slightly.

To release the pose, unclasp the feet and stretch out the legs.

5. *Gomukhāsana*: Cow-Faced Pose

Legs: From a seated position with the legs extended in front, bend the knees and bring the soles of the feet to the floor. Draw the left leg under the right, bringing the left heel to the outside of the right buttock. Bring the right leg over the left, attempting to line up the knees. Place the right heel to the outside of the left buttock.

Arms: Avoid slumping throughout. Raise the right arm overhead and bend the elbow, bringing the forearm behind the back. Align the palm of the right hand with the spine. Draw the left arm behind the back and work toward holding hands together. (If the hands are too far apart, use a strap or cloth.) Align the left forearm with the spine if comfortable.

To exit, unclasp the hands, uncross the legs, and return the soles of the feet to the floor. Reverse the arms and legs.

6. Cat / Cow Pose

Come onto the hands and knees with the knees below the hips. Roll the tailbone down and under while arching the back upward, and draw the chin toward the chest. Then raise the tailbone up, release the abdomen downward, and bring the chest and chin forward. Repeat several times. The movements may be coordinated with the breath. Exhale into cat position and inhale into cow position.

To exit, return the spine to a neutral position.

Cat 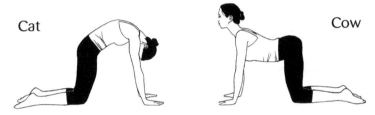 Cow

7. *Setu Bandhāsana*: Bridge Pose

Lie on the back with the knees bent, and place the feet on the floor so that the ankles are under the knees and as wide apart as the hips. Check that the neck feels comfortable. Remove any hair or clothing that might cause discomfort. Place the arms alongside the body, palms facing down. Pressing into the feet, slowly lift the hips upward and the chest toward the chin.

To exit, slowly lower down vertebra by vertebra.

Yoga Mudrā: Yogic Seal

Technique: Sit in whatever cross-legged position is comfortable with the spine erect, eyes closed. Bring the hands behind the back and take hold of one wrist. Inhale and lengthen the spine. Exhale and hinge forward from the hips. Come forward as far as is comfortable. Relax the head and shoulders. Relax the breath. Bring the awareness within.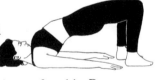

Inhale and very slowly raise the head, lengthen the spine and come up to a seated position. Keeping the eyes closed, return the hands to the knees. Take a couple of slow, deep breaths, and sit quietly for a moment, observing how you feel.

Time: Once for 30 seconds.

Benefits: Soothes the nervous system by helping to balance the parasympathetic and sympathetic parts of the autonomic nervous system. May aid in the relief of many abdominal disorders, including constipation. Energetically begins the transition to the more subtle aspects of the Integral Yoga class.

Yoga Nidrā: Yogic Sleep or Deep Relaxation

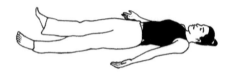

Technique: Lie on the back in *śavāsana* with the feet about shoulder distance apart and the arms a few inches from the body, palms up, and close the eyes. Raise, squeeze and then abruptly relax each part of the body in this order: right leg, left leg, right arm, left arm, buttocks, abdomen, chest, shoulders, neck and then face. With the body remaining still, check over each part mentally. If you find any tension, mentally release it. Now watch the breath, letting it be completely relaxed. Then begin to watch the thoughts of the mind. Feel that you are the witness—not the body or mind—the True Self. Remain this way for at least five minutes.

Come out of the relaxation slowly by imagining fresh energy entering each part of the body from the head downward. Wiggle the fingers and toes, roll the arms and legs from side to side and stretch. Slowly sit up.

Time: 15 minutes total.

Benefits: A great stress-reduction technique. Allows the benefits of the Hatha Yoga session to be assimilated, and helps to calm the mind.

Prāṇāyāma: Breathing Practice

Prāṇāyāma helps to burn out toxins that may have been released into the bloodstream by the āsanas. Just as the āsanas give us control over the physical body, prāṇāyāma helps us to gain control over the prāṇa, or vital life energy, and ultimately over the mind.

Dīrgha Śwāsam: Deep Breathing

Technique: Sit in a cross-legged posture with spine erect. Breathe slowly and deeply in three parts. To begin the practice, exhale fully through the nose. To inhale, expand the abdomen first, and then feel the rib cage lift and expand, and finally the collarbones rise. Exhale from the upper chest, feeling the collarbones lower, then relax the lower ribs and gently draw in the abdomen to empty the lungs.

Close the eyes and continue, letting the parts blend one into the next, so the breath is one continuous, smooth flow. Breathe slowly and deeply. End with an exhalation after several rounds.

Time: A minimum of several minutes. Can be practiced any time during the day.

Benefits: By breathing this way you utilize the full capacity of the lungs, taking in several times more oxygen and prāṇa than in normal, shallow breathing. Calms the mind. Forms the foundation for all other prāṇāyāma practices.

Kapālabhāti: Skull Shining Breath

Technique: Forcefully expel the breath through the nostrils by contracting the abdomen. Then relax the abdomen allowing the breath to return without effort. Have about 15 expulsions in rapid succession, then exhale deeply, enjoy one three-part breath and return to normal breathing.

Time: 3 rounds with 15–30 expulsions. Gradually increase number of expulsions per round and number of rounds.

Benefits: Cleans the nāḍis (the subtle energy channels) in the skull. Burns out excess mucus that causes sinus problems and allergies. Stimulates digestive organs. Clears the mind.

Nāḍi Śuddhi: Nerve Cleansing Breath

Technique: Make a gentle fist with the right hand. Extend the thumb, ring finger and little finger, leaving the two middle fingers tucked into the palm. Bring the fist in front of the nose. Inhale into both nostrils. Close the right nostril with 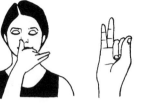 the thumb and slowly exhale through the left nostril using the Yogic deep breathing. Inhale into the left, close it with the last two fingers and exhale through the right.

When you get accustomed to this, establish a count whereby your exhalation is twice as long as your inhalation. For example, if you inhale counting "*OM* 1, *OM* 2," exhale counting "*OM* 1, *OM* 2, *OM* 3, *OM* 4." Gradually increase the count without changing this ratio. End with an exhalation through the right nostril.

Time: About 3 minutes to start and gradually increasing to 10 or more complete rounds.

Benefits: Brings lightness of body, mental alertness, good appetite, proper digestion and sound sleep. Calms and cleanses the nervous system and helps focus the mind. Balances the left and right hemispheres of the brain. Good preparation for meditation.

Chanting and Meditation

Having made the body and mind calm and relaxed through the *Hatha Yoga* practice, this is an excellent opportunity to practice at least a few minutes of meditation. First you may wish to stretch out the legs if they feel cramped and then resume your cross-legged position. To further concentrate and elevate the mind you may chant a *mantra* such as "*OM Śāntih*," "*Hari Om*," or "*Om*" aloud for a few minutes. Then begin to repeat the *mantra* silently, feeling the vibration. Another form of meditation would be to simply watch the breath. Or you can combine watching the breath with repeating the *mantra*. Keep the body perfectly still during this time and feel the peace. You may finish your practice with the following prayers:

OM Śāntiḥ Music (OM Peace)

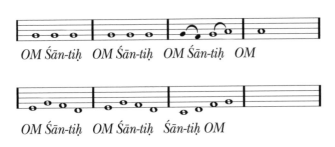

OM Śān-tiḥ   OM Śān-tiḥ   OM Śān-tiḥ   OM

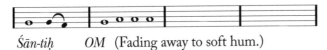

OM Śān-tiḥ   OM Śān-tiḥ   Śān-tiḥ   OM

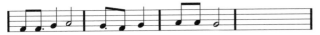

Śān-tiḥ   OM   (Fading away to soft hum.)

Closing Chants Music

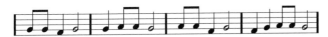

A-sat-o Mā   /Sad Ga-ma-ya/Ta-ma-so Mā/Jyo-tir Ga-ma-ya
Lead us from unreal to Real; Lead us from darkness to Light;

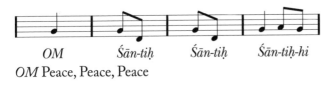

Mṛi-tyor Mā/   Ām-ṛi-tam/   Ga-ma-ya
Lead us from the fear of death to the knowledge of Immortality.

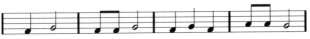

OM   Śān-tiḥ   Śān-tiḥ   Śān-tiḥ-hi
OM Peace, Peace, Peace

Lo-kāḥ   Sa-mas-tāḥ   Su-khi-no   Bha-van-tu
May the entire universe be filled with peace and joy, love and light.

Jai Śri Sadguru Mahārāj Kī–Jai!
Victory to that Light–Victory!

To learn more about the philosophy behind, and the power within, *Hatha Yoga*, I would recommend Pandit Usharbudh Arya's *Philosophy of Hatha Yoga*. In this compact little text, Arya writes: "In a single *Hatha* session, you pass through the entire cycle of reincarnation, pass through the entire cycle of having been a camel and having been an amoeba, and the entire cycle of creation, preservation and destruction. Every day, creation of a mood, preservation of that mood and removal of that mood to something else can be accomplished at your will. A dancer will tell you that true dance comes from the mood. You create the mood and then become that." According to him, if we have the courage to confront the discomfort that we feel when we attempt to establish discipline of body and mind, then *Hatha Yoga* serves as *tapasya*, literally "burning." *Hatha Yoga*, says Arya, is actually a burning of *karma*. So, if you'd like to escape from the prison of continual birth and rebirth, *Hatha Yoga* may be the route that awaits you.

Brahmacharya (Celibacy)

At the *ashram*, monks and single people practice celibacy, *brahmacharya* in Sanskrit. In his commentary on Patanjali's Yoga *Sutras*, Gurudev talks about *tapas* as an austerity, whereby one accepts pain—whether physical or emotional—as purification. He emphasizes, though, that while austerities are an important aid to self-discipline (*tapas* also refers to self-discipline), they should never become self-torture, like lying on a bed of nails or keeping one arm raised in the air so that the arm gets thinner and thinner until it finally decays, extreme types of physical austerities practiced by some *sadhus*, or ascetics, in India and in other Eastern cultures. Gurudev further explains that these types of harsh austerities are not aids to spiritual growth; rather, they are obstacles. In fact, Lord Krishna calls those ascetics demons, because they disturb the pure Self that dwells within their bodies, and he classifies the true austerities of the body as worship, purity, straightforwardness, celibacy and non-injury. Of course, some people might consider celibacy, *brahmahcarya*, to be an unsuitable austerity, at least for them. But *brahmacharya* means control or moderation. It doesn't mean suppression of sexuality. That's why householders don't normally renounce sexual activity, but they enjoy it in moderation.

On the other hand, for such individuals as monks who have chosen the path of renunciation, spiritual seekers who choose to renounce sexual activity for a long or short period of time as part of their program of self-discipline, or prisoners who are expected to remain celibate while they are incarcerated, *brahmacharya* also means celibacy.

What's important to understand, though, is that *brahmacharya* as celibacy does not mean *suppression* of sexual desire or sexual force. Rather, it means *sublimation*. Suppression of desire only strengthens that desire. Constantly trying to overcome the desire, we become more and more attached to it, and, invariably, we become restless and angry. But if we fill our minds with sublime thoughts by meditating, chanting, repeating a *mantra*, praying, studying scriptures, contemplating the pure, sexless Self, then, as Gurudev assures us, the sexual desire "will be devitalized by the withdrawal of the mind."

Moreover, through *Hatha Yoga*, the body itself can be enlisted to support the practice of *brahmacharya*. Fundamentally, all the *Hatha* poses can help to control sexual desire and the sexual force. However, there are specific poses that facilitate and support the practice of *brahmacharya*: Lotus Pose (*Padmasana*); Accomplished Pose (*Siddhasana*); Heroic Pose (*Veerasana*); Head-to-Knee Pose (*Janusirshasana*); Forward-Bending Pose (*Paschimothanasana*); Head Stand (*Sirshasana*); Bound Lotus Pose (*Baddha Padmasana*); the *bandhas*, or locks (these should be undertaken only with the guidance of a well-trained and experienced Yoga instructor): Chin Lock (*Jalandhra Bandha*), Anus Lock (*Mula Bandha*) and the Stomach Lift (*Uddhiyana Bandha*); Alternate Nostril Breathing (*Nadi Suddhi*). Finally, one of the most powerful techniques that can be employed to establish and maintain celibacy is *Savasana*, the Corpse Pose, because during *Savasana* the mind becomes a spiritual instrument. It's especially useful to do *Savasana* before sleep.

Another factor that has an impact on celibacy is diet. If you're planning to practice or are already practicing celibacy, it's important to avoid foods that stimulate the system. Thus, garlic, onions and spicy foods should be eliminated from the diet.

In *Practice of Brahmacharya*, one of his more than 200 books on Yoga philosophy and practices and spirituality in general, Swami Sivananda catalogs the many profound benefits of the practice of *brahmacharya*:

Practice of *brahmacharya* gives good health, inner strength, peace of mind and long life. It invigorates the mind and nerves. It helps to conserve physical and mental energy. It augments memory, will force and brain power. It bestows tremendous strength, vigor and vitality. Strength and fortitude are obtained . . . . He who is established in *brahmacharya* will have lustrous eyes, a sweet voice and a beautiful complexion."

As both a physician and a renunciate, Swami Sivananda's words are based on first-hand experience. His dynamism, charisma and enormous capacity for work (which he saw as worship) attest to the efficacy of *brahmacharya* and a life devoted to selfless service.

Ashram Diet

At the *ashram*, we follow a strict vegetarian diet; that is, we don't eat meat, fish, or eggs. Some people choose to follow a vegan diet, eliminating all animal products, including dairy products and honey. Some follow a raw food diet for long or short periods of time. If you're interested in starting a raw food diet, it's best not to eat too much at one time, one, because there's so much energy in raw food that you don't need to take in as much as when you're eating cooked food, which loses a lot of the energy and nutrition during cooking, and, two, because your system is used to digesting cooked food, so it will find it harder to digest only raw food for awhile. Also, we don't eat lots of onions or garlic (except if we're using garlic for medicinal purposes–it's a natural antibiotic), which are stimulants that might make the mind restless and less fit for meditation, nor do we use very spicy foods or much sugar for the same reason. With respect to daily meals, the yogic diet consists of a light breakfast (fruit, yogurt, or cereal) and a light supper (fruit, yogurt, cereal, salad, soup). The main meal is at lunchtime.

According to the yogic teachings, food isn't linked only to the body, but it also is directly connected to the mind. According to these teachings, we're not physically constructed to eat meat. We can't see well at night like the animals who are natural hunters. Our teeth are flat, not hooked, and our tongues are soft, not rough like those animals that eat flesh. We can't digest meat in our natural state—our intestines are much, much longer than those of meat-eating animals, so meat sits in the intestines, and it takes a long time before waste matter is eliminated, whereas flesh-eating animals have short intestines, so that meat is quickly digested and the waste eliminated in a shorter time. Moreover, the purine that is contained in meat converts into cholesterol, which can cause serious health problems.

Of course, dairy products also come from animals and are not always easy to digest, especially for people who are lactose intolerant. But milk is considered to be different from flesh, because it's taken from the mother and not from the mother's flesh. Additionally, according to the yogic teachings, milk has a special quality; it's a *sattvic* food, meaning that it's balanced and calming, and it doesn't have the concentrated fat that's found in meat; however, if we eat too much dairy, it becomes hard to digest and causes phlegm.

From the spiritual perspective, yogis don't eat meat, because they are practicing *ahimsa*, non-violence, and want to cause as little pain as possible. But plants also have consciousness, so how can we rationalize eating them? Don't we hurt them, too? According to Gurudev, yes, we probably do hurt them when we eat them, but the consciousness in a plant is less sensitive; it's like dreaming. So, the goal is that we cause the least pain as possible in our daily life. Of course, if, for some reason, you have no choice but to eat meat to survive, then you must do it if there's nothing else available. In such a situation, you can at least feel grateful to the animal whose life was sacrificed.

Spiritual Diary

Another valuable tool for spiritual growth and transformation, one that many people use at the *ashram*, is the spiritual diary. The spiritual diary gives you the opportunity to develop self-discipline and willpower, to confront your strengths and weaknesses in all areas, and to increase self-knowledge.

To begin your spiritual diary, you can make a few resolves. It's better to make resolves that you have a good chance of keeping. Give yourself a break, and don't try the impossible, at least not at first. For example, you might make a resolve to get up early to do spiritual practices, meditate regularly, for at least fifteen minutes every day, do *Hatha Yoga* three times a week, maintain silence once a week, do physical exercises for fifteen minutes every day, read from a scripture every day, refrain from using aggressive language, refrain from eating junk food, stay on a vegetarian or vegan diet for a certain period of time, fast once a month, or write in your spiritual diary every day. You get the picture. Write down your resolves in the beginning of the diary and then, each day, record your successes and failures.

The format of the diary can take any form you wish. You can use a book with blank pages, a pad, or any other type of journal. You can make a list of questions to answer, like: When did I get out of bed this morning? Did I do *Hatha Yoga*? If so, for how long? How long did I meditate? Did I spend any time doing spiritual practices? How was my attitude toward others? Did I lose my temper? You might prefer to have a sheet with columns, listing spiritual practices, dates and times of practice and checks to indicate whether you practiced or not.

The spiritual diary serves as an instrument of self-evaluation. It promotes self-discipline and opens the door to self-knowledge.

It goes without saying that following an *ashram* schedule and a yogic lifestyle in prison will present greater challenges than following them outside of prison: narrower dietetic choices, a less supportive environment, less freedom to create one's own schedule, maybe not so much room to do the practices, and probably less privacy, etc. On the other hand, as I've alluded to throughout this book, compared to people living in the larger society, individuals who are incarcerated have fewer day-to-day responsibilities, so they have more time and energy to devote to spiritual studies and practices if they have the inclination and the will to do so. And to press my point, may I remind you of an old maxim: Obstacles are stepping stones to success.

Epilogue: One Step at a Time

By the practice of the limbs of Yoga, the impurities dwindle away and
there dawns the light of wisdom, leading to discriminative discernment.
—Yoga Sutras of Patanjali, *Book 2, Sutra 28*

Just the other day, I heard on my local National Public Radio station that many of our nation's prisons are overcrowded and understaffed. Obviously, the challenges associated with the operation of such a large prison system are numerous and complex, and, as with any huge institution, it would be unrealistic to anticipate simple and speedy reforms. On the other hand, at least as important as the issue of prison reform is the subject of prisoner reform.

As I've sought to illustrate in this book, prisoners who have been provided with the means to transform their thinking and their behavior from the negative to the positive and from the destructive to the productive are able to thrive in the most adverse conditions. Moreover, these people have a powerful, transforming effect on others. I've seen it happen before and I'm seeing it happen now. In fact, I've recently been contacted by a prisoner who has been serving a two-year sentence and is about to be released from a nearby correctional facility. He is enthusiastic about starting a prison *ashram* program that includes Yoga and meditation. With the support of a Buddhist friend on the outside, this fellow began studying Buddhist philosophy and practicing Yoga and meditation, and he read Bo Lozoff's book. He gained so much benefit from his studies and practices—improved health, self-knowledge, peace of mind—that he felt compelled to share what he was learning and experiencing with some interested fellow inmates. Now, he and a few other inmates (who have also begun corresponding with me) are keenly interested in working to establish a program at their facility based on Yoga and meditation, and they've asked me to be their sponsor and instructor. Obviously, my time in prison is not over.

I have recently received my new volunteer identification card and have been informed that the men who are interested in such a program are being interviewed. I'm really excited that I'm about to embark on a new prison experience. I know that there will be many challenges. All bureaucratic institutions abound in rules and regulations and one can imagine that in such a high security environment, prisons rely on many policies that test one's patience and endurance. The way I look at it, the process of organizing a prison Yoga program, for all concerned, will be like the practice of walking meditation: one slow step at a time, with the mind focused on each step, each moment, as we move closer and closer to the liberating force of Self-knowledge.

Resources

Books

Pandit Usharbudh Arya ((1981). *Philosophy of Hatha Yoga.* Honesdale: The Himalayan International Institute of Yoga Science and Philosophy.

Divine Life Society *(1985). Sivananda, Biography of a Modern Sage (Life and Works of Swami Sivananda, vol. 1). Sivanandanagar, India: Divine Life Society Publications.*

Trisha Lamb (2006). *Yoga in Prison.* A comprehensive bibliography of books, articles and videos about Yoga and meditation programs in correctional institutions, treatment facilities and healthcare centers. Prescott, AZ: International Association of Yoga Therapists (IAYT).

Lucy Lidell et al (1983). *The Sivananda Companion to Yoga.* New York: Simon & Schuster Inc.

Bo Lozoff (1985). *We're All Doing Time: A Guide to Getting Free.* Durham: Prison- Ashram Project.

Swami Rama, Rudolph Ballentine, M.D., Alan Hymes, M.D ((1981). *Science of Breath.* Honesdale: The Himalayan International Institute of Yoga Science and Philosophy.

Swami Satchidananda: Apostle of Peace. Eds. Sita Bordow et al (1986). Buckingham: Integral Yoga Publications.

Swami Satchidananda (1970). *Integral Yoga Hatha.* New York: Holt, Rinehart and Winston.

Swami Satchidananda (1988). *The Living Gita.* Buckingham: Integral Yoga Publications.

Swami Satchidananda (1975). *Meditation.* Pomfret Center: Integral Yoga Publications.

Swami Satchidananda, translation and commentary (1978). *The Yoga Sutras of Patanjali.* Buckingham: Integral Yoga Publications.

Swami Satchidananda (1978). *To Know Your Self.* Ed. Philip Mandelkorn. Buckingham: Integral Yoga Publications.

Swami Satyananda Saraswati (1998). *Yoga Nidra*. Bihar: Yoga Publications Trust.

The Yoga Sutras of Patanjali (2004). Translation and commentary by Sri Swami Satchidananda. Buckingham: Integral Yoga Publications

Swami Sivananda (1975). Concentration and Meditation. Shivanandanagar: The Divine Life Society.

Swami Sivananda (1974). Mind, Its Mysteries and Control. Shivanandanagar: The Divine Life Society.

Swami Vivekananda (1982). *Raja-Yoga*. New York: Ramakrishna-Vivekananda Center.

Articles

Janaki, Sannyasi (1999, November). Benefits of Yoga for Prison Inmates. *Yoga Magazine*. yogamag.net

Wikipedia. Prisons in the United States. wikipedia.org

Pew Charitable Trusts (2007, February 14). Public Safety, Public Spending: Forecasting America's Prison Population: 2007-2011. Prisons in the United States. Prison Growth Could Cost up to $27.5 Billion Over Next 5 Years: New Report Projects National and State-by-State Prison Populations in 2011. *Public Safety Performance Project* pewpublicsafety.org

Krisberg, B. & Marchionna, Susan (2006, April). FOCUS, Views from the National Council on Crime and Delinquency (NCCD). nccd-crc.org

Penal Reform International (2007). Penal Reform Briefing No. 2. penalreform.org

Think Quest (2003, August 6). The United States Prison System: A Glimpse Behind the Bars. library.thinkquest.org

Center on Juvenile and Criminal Justice (2002). America's One Million Nonviolent Prisoners. cjcj.org

The Natural Law Party. Crime. natural-law.org

Author's name omitted by request (2001, Nov. 30). Prison Industry vs. Prisoner Rehabilitation in Florida. prisonerlife.com (an open and uncensored forum networking prisoners, prisons and the world).

Commission on Safety and Abuse in Prison. www.infoplease.com

Mithra (1971). Jail Yoga. *Integral Yoga Magazine*, Light 2, Ray 11 & 12.

Cohen, Kanniah (1972). Community Service: Danbury Federal Prison. *Integral Yoga Magazine*, Light 3, Ray 14.

Satchidananda, Swami (1972). Swamiji Speaks at Danbury Prison. *Integral Yoga Magazine*, Light 3, Ray 15.

Dorji, Brahmachari (1972). Community Service: Lorton Complex. *Integral Yoga Magazine.*

de Sachy, Rev. Kumari (1997, Spring). Prison Yoga. *Integral Yoga Magazine*, pp. 18-29.

Mercadante, Linda. Morris Inmates Turn To Yoga. *Satchidananda Ashram Archives.*

Hallett, Bruce. Heaven in Prison: Yogi Visits Inmates. *Satchidananda Ashram Archives.*

O'Brien, Tim. Jail Yoga Class May Lose Funds. *Satchidananda Ashram Archives.*

Shihab, Aziz (September 26, 1973). Be Good, Do Good, Swami Advises. *San Antonio News.*

Pozzi, Vimala (2000, Summer). Yoga at Bon Air Juvenile Correctional Center. *The OM News*, p. 7.

Boehn, Caryn (1999, Fall). Yoga in Bon Air. *The OM News*, p. 5.

Dunn, Chris (1999, Fall). Teaching Yoga in Prisons. *The OM News*, p. 5.

Recordings

Swami Satchidananda. (1973, September 20). Swami Satchidananda speaking at Soledad Prison [CD]. Buckingham: Shakticom/Satchidananda Ashram.

Swami Satchidananda (1973, September 21). Swami Satchidananda speaking at Deuel Vocational Institute [CD]. Buckingham: Shakticom/Satchidananda Ashram.

Swami Satchidananda. (1976, July 20). Swami Satchidananda speaking at the Dallas Detention Center [CD]. Buckingham: Shakticom/Satchidananda Ashram.

Swami Satchidananda (1996, August 5). Swami Satchidananda speaking at the Buckingham Correctional Center [CD]. Buckingham: Shakticom/Satchidananda Ashram.

Rev. Jaganath Carrera. (1991). *Prison Yoga* [CD]. Buckingham: Shakticom/Satchidananda Ashram.

DVDs

Ariel, Eilona & Menahemi, Ayelet (Directors). (1997). *Doing Time, Doing Vipassana* [Motion picture]. Israel: Karuna Films

Connelley, Sean & Newton, Katie (Director). (2004). *Going Within, Yoga in the San Francisco County Jail*. United States: Oakland Tribune.

Programs

Satchidananda Prison Project
Satchidananda Ashram-Yogaville
108 Yogaville Way, Buckingham, Virginia 23921 USA
Tel: 434-969-3121 ext 116
programs@iyiva.org / www.iyiva.org

The Prison Project
c/o SYDA Foundation
PO Box 99140, Emeryville, CA 94662 USA
Tel: 510-898-2771
PrisonProject@syaoakland.org
www.oaklandsyda.org

Bihar School of Yoga's Prison Project
Secretary, Bihar School of Yoga
Ganga Darshan, Fort, Munger, Bihar 811201 India
Tel: +91 (0)6344 222430 / Fax: +91 (0)6344 220169
www.yogavision.net

Prison-Ashram Project
c/o Human Kindness Foundation
PO Box 61619, Durham, NC 27715 USA
Tel: 919-383-5160
www.humankindness.org

Insight Prison Project
805 Fourth Street, Suite 3, San Rafael, CA 94901 USA
Tel: 415-459-9800 / Fax: 415-459-9801
info@InsightPrisonProject.org / www.insightprisonproject.org

Living Yoga
P.O. Box 69065, Portland, OR 97230 USA
Tel: 503-546-1269
www.living-yoga.org

Rural Rejuvenation Prison Outreach ("Inner Freedom for the
Imprisoned" Yoga programs)
c/o Isha Institute of Inner Sciences
951 Isha Lane, McMinnville, TN 37110 USA
Tel: 931-668-1900
usa@ishafoundation.org / www.ruralrejuvenation.org

Tamil Nadu Prison Department–Reformation of Prisoners
c/o Director General of Prisons
CMDA Tower-II, No.1, Gandhi Irwin Road, Egmore,
Chennai 600 008 India
Tel: +91 44 (0)28521306
www.prisons.tn.nic.in

Prison Dharma Network
PO Box 4623, Boulder CO 80306 USA
Tel: 303-544-5923
info@prisondharmanetwork.org / www.prisondharmanetwork.org

The Lionheart Foundation
PO Box 170115, Boston, MA 02117 USA
Tel: 781-444-6667 / Fax: 781-444-6855
questions@lionheart.org / www.lionheart.org

The Zone: A Teen Center for the Mind, Body, & Heart
c/o The Lineage Project
PO Box 4668 #8375
New York, NY 10163
beth@lineageproject.org / www.lineageproject.org

Yoga Outreach
PO Box 29157, Vancouver, BC, V6J 5C2, Canada
Tel: 604-505-7547
kyira@yogaoutreach.com / www.yogaoutreach.com

Freeing the Human Spirit
Box 65142, 358 Danforth Ave., Toronto, ON, M4K 3Z2, Canada
Tel: 416-285-4872
freeingspirit@rogers.com / www.freeingspirit.com

Buddhist Peace Fellowship Prison Project "Prison Meditation Groups"
(research by Connie Kassor)
PO Box 3470, Berkeley, CA 94703 USA
Tel: 510-655-6169 / Fax: 510-655-1369
membership@bpf.org / www.bpf.org

Free Books for Prisoners Programs

Books Behind Bars (A project of the Quest Institute)
c/o Quest Bookshop

619 W Main St, Charlottesville, VA 22903 USA
Tel: 434-295-3377
www.thequestbookshop.com

Books to Prisoners
c/o Left Bank Books
92 Pike Street, Box A, Seattle, WA 98101 USA
Tel: 206-622-0195
bookstoprisoners@cs.com / www.bookstoprisoners.net

Olympia Books to Prisoners
P.O. Box 912, Olympia, WA 98507 USA
Tel: 360-352-5460
btpoly@2resist.ca / www.btpolympia.org

Portland Books to Prisoners
1112 NE Morton, Portland, OR 97211
pdxbookstoprisoners@riseup.net / www.bookstooregonprisoners.org

Bellingham Books to Prisoners
P.O. Box 1254, Bellingham, WA 98227
Tel: 360-733-9099
bhambtp@yahoo.com

UC BUC Books to Prisoners
Box 515, Urbana, IL 61803
www.books2prisoners.org

Wisconsin Books to Prisoners Project
c/o Madison Infoshop
1019 Williamson St. #B, Madison, WI 53703
Tel: 608-262-9036
wisconsinbookstoprisoners@yahoo.com

Prison Book Program
c/o Lucy Parsons Bookstore
1306 Hancock Street, Suite 100, Quincy, MA 02169
Tel: 617-423-3298 (no collect calls)
info@prisonbookprogram.org // www.prisonbookprogram.org

Note: There are many more programs than listed below. Almost every city, and certainly every state, has organizations that provide free prison books. Search online for "free books for prisoners" and add the city/state for further listings.

For an extensive, though not updated, list go to: www.freewebs.com/books4prisoners/resourcelinks.htm.

Sri Swami Satchidananda was one of the first Yoga masters to bring the classical Yoga tradition to the West. He taught Yoga postures to Americans, introduced them to meditation, a vegetarian diet and more compassionate lifestyle.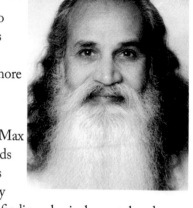

During this period of cultural awakening, iconic pop artist Peter Max and a small circle of his artist friends beseeched the Swami to extend his brief stop in New York City so they could learn from him the secret of finding physical, mental and spiritual health, peace and enlightenment.

Three years later, he led some half a million American youth in chanting OM, when he delivered the official opening remarks at the 1969 Woodstock Music and Art Festival and he became known as "the Woodstock Guru."

The distinctive teachings he brought with him blend the physical discipline of Yoga, the spiritual philosophy of Vedantic literature and the interfaith ideals he pioneered.

These techniques and concepts influenced a generation and spawned a Yoga culture that is flourishing today. Today, over twenty million Americans practice Yoga as a means for managing stress, promoting health, slowing down the aging process and creating a more meaningful life.

The teachings of Swami Satchidananda have spread into the mainstream and thousands of people now teach Yoga. Integral Yoga is the foundation for Dr. Dean Ornish's landmark work in reversing heart disease and Dr. Michael Lerner's noted Commonweal Cancer Help program.

Today many Integral Yoga Institutes, teaching centers and certified teachers throughout the United States and abroad offer classes and training programs in all aspects of Integral Yoga.

In 1979, Sri Swamiji was inspired to establish Satchidananda Ashram–Yogaville. Based on his teachings, it is a place where people of different faiths and backgrounds can come to realize their essential oneness.

One of the focal points of Yogaville is the Light Of Truth Universal Shrine (LOTUS). This unique interfaith shrine honors the Spirit that unites all the world religions, while celebrating their diversity. People from all over the world come there to meditate and pray.

Over the years, Sri Swamiji received many honors for his public service, including the Juliet Hollister Interfaith Award presented at the United Nations and in 2002 the U Thant Peace Award.

In addition, he served on the advisory boards of many Yoga, world peace and interfaith organizations. He is the author of many books on Yoga and is the subject of the documentary, *Living Yoga: The life and teachings of Swami Satchidananda.*

In 2002, he entered *Mahasamadhi* (a God-realized soul's conscious final exit from the body).

For more information, visit: www.swamisatchidananda.org

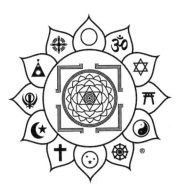

Designed by Swami Satchidananda, the All Faiths Yantra is an external image representing the central tenet of Swami Satchidananda's teaching: "Truth is one, paths are many." Symbols in the petals, clockwise from top: Faiths Still Unknown, Hinduism, Judaism, Shinto, Taoism, Buddhism, Other Known Faiths, Christianity, Islam, Sikhism, Traditional African Faiths, Native American Faiths.

About the Author

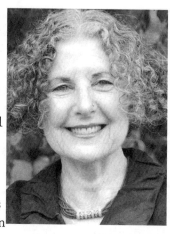

Rev. Sandra Kumari de Sachy has been studying and practicing Integral Yoga since 1980. She became a certified Integral Yoga teacher in 1981 and was ordained as an Integral Yoga minister in 1995.

She has taught Hatha Yoga, Yoga philosophy and meditation in colleges and universities, in Yoga centers and in prison, and she continues to teach.

She has a Masters degree in English Literature and a doctorate in English Education from Rutgers University and has taught both English and Yoga in colleges and universities in the US and in France.

One of the most transforming experiences in her life was teaching Creative Writing and Yoga at the Buckingham Correctional Center in Dillwyn, Virginia.

Rev. de Sachy lives with her husband at Satchidananda Ashram-Yogaville in Buckingham, Virginia.